EATING DISORDERS:
Managing Problems with Food

Paul Haskew, Ed.D.
Psychologist
University Health Services
University of Connecticut
Storrs, CT 06268

Cynthia H. Adams, Ph.D.
Associate Professor
School of Allied Health Professions
University of Connecticut
Storrs, CT 06268

Glencoe Publishing Company
Mission Hills, California

Send all inquiries to:
Glencoe Publishing Company
15319 Chatsworth Street
Mission Hills, California 91345

Printed in the United States of America

ISBN 0-02-685630-1

1 2 3 4 5   92 91 90 89 88

Diane Beasley, Cover and Interior Design
Creative Slides and Advertising, Charts and Graphs
Llyn Hunter, Cartoonist

EATING DISORDERS:
Managing Problems with Food

CONTENTS

Have you heard or read about the terms *anorexia* and *bulimia?* Do these words make you think of a rare illness suffered by some unlucky few? If so, you are wrong.

Have you gone through periods of being concerned, almost to the point of obsession, about your weight? Do you feel ashamed of every ounce of fat on your body? Have you tried a number of different diet programs? If so, this book is for you.

A peculiar obsession has arisen in Western society. A fear of fat and a desire to be thin have overcome rational thought in the minds of millions. The consequences of our obsession with thinness are needless misery for many. And, as always happens when people want what they cannot have, it has handsomely enriched opportunists who trade on such fads and fears.

Fashion has declared that gaunt and bony is beautiful. Medicine has declared (with inappropriate firmness and insufficient hard facts) that obesity is hazardous to our health. Women have found that a feminine fullness handicaps their struggle to compete as equals with men. The postwar baby boomers have reached middle age and have begun to experience "middle-aged spread."

Upset because we no longer feel or look 25, millions of us have taken up the battle against fat. Meanwhile, the food industry has learned to employ the most persuasive advertising techniques to market low-quality, high-profit, high-calorie manufactured foods to a populace that has less time and less opportunity to prepare nutritious meals from unprocessed foodstuffs.

Finally, and perhaps most important of all, there is a widespread illusion that the concept of all men being created equal means that everyone, but especially every woman, has an equal opportunity and an equal responsibility to fit the current norms for acceptable appearance. To assert that not everyone can or should be thin may be to risk being labeled sexist or undemocratic, but that's exactly what we're doing.

The impact of powerful social pressures on young people to be thin has been predictably calamitous. Children in grade school can be heard chatting about the latest fad diet. With innocent daring and a sincere desire to fit in, they begin to battle with their appetites in an unwitting attempt to stem their normal development. In our high schools today, anorexia is rampant, and self-starvation has come to be a common expression of strength and status. Even punitive and self-abusive exercising is perceived as a minimal response to the need to avoid getting fat.

Adults, too—with barely greater sophistication—furiously diet, exercise, and medicate themselves in a struggle to achieve or maintain a thin figure.

Few, if any, of these people realize that in resolving to reduce their widths, they are taking on adversaries of formidable strength; namely, their own minds and bodies. Some will succeed in "disciplining" themselves. Others will come to recognize that they are losing the battle and will seek a compromise. Many will engage in periodic battles with fat, using books and programs that help them lose a few pounds now and then, only to gain them back a month or two later. The rest will become casualties: victims to greater or lesser degrees of compulsive eating, bulimia, anorexia, self-induced vomiting, laxative abuse, anxiety, depression, isolation, self-hatred, and weight gain.

Our purpose is to present, in a concise and readable format, enough details about this epidemic of appetite disorders to enable informed persons, students, educators, concerned parents, and health professionals to understand, relieve, and even prevent them. In this one volume we address both eating disorders and obesity, which we see as separate but related topics.

This book presents the knowledge we have gained through the work of others, through our own research, and, most important, through the lessons our students have taught us. Although the examples we present are fictional, all are based on behaviors we have observed and statements we have heard. They provide an insider's view of the harsh struggles, and sometimes remarkable outcomes, of our work with a small part of a national epidemic.

Clinical experience and the research literature have convinced us that our approach is psychologically and physiologically sound, and that it provides eating-disordered persons with new ways of thinking and acting that allow them to regain their health, strength, and self-respect.

In preparing this book, we have been greatly helped by the support and encouragement of our colleagues in the University Health Service and School of Allied Health Professions at the University of Connecticut. We would especially like to thank Dr. Peter Jones and Dr. Joseph Nowinski for their thoughtful reviews and comments, and our editors Luan Corrigan and Kathy Wolter for their invaluable help in creating a readable manuscript. Our greatest debt of gratitude, however, is owed to the many clients and students whose insights pointed the ways to recovery and helped generate the ideas that have in turn enabled us to help others.

APPETITE DISORDERS
The Dieter's Disease

This chapter will help you:

1. Describe the relationship between cultural pressures and dieting for cosmetic change.
2. Describe the relationship between dieting and appetite or eating disorders (pathorexia).
3. Define pathorexia.
4. Understand that obesity is not a disease.

◆

"It's not that I want to be one of the crowd, but I do want to be what the crowd thinks is best."

The quest for beauty surely began at the dawn of society, and the search for relief from unfashionable fatness may be almost as old. The Romans' use of vomitoriums and the Victorians' inclusion of live tapeworms in their diet are two of the more bizarre, though probably more successful, techniques that have been employed in that pursuit. A third technique—dieting—has also always been known and used.

Jenny

Jenny always knew she was fat, and her weight was always a problem. For example, when her preschool ballet teacher assigned her to the second row in the chorus and gave her the lead in "The Teddy Bears Picnic," she contented herself in the belief that there is a place in the sun for everyone. In grade school, she enjoyed being the first in her class to fit into grownup clothes. In junior high, when her bust filled quickly to splendid dimensions, she felt mature and female. In those years, being fat was a disadvantage but not a disaster.

At 15, Jenny's world fell apart. By then, it seemed, she had become everything nobody wanted to be. The phone stopped ringing, her friends paired off without her, and she began to feel like a leper.

Jenny's mother knew what had happened; so did her dad. Fat people themselves, they had known rejection, too. Although they ached to be of help, Jenny's eyes blazed with blame and disgust whenever they tried to talk to her. They watched helplessly as she withdrew, clinging to a strict diet.

Because dieting is often successful in causing an initial weight loss, any reluctance to diet counts heavily against fat people in public opinion. In addition, the assumption that obesity is the result of gluttony and lack of self-control has created an almost universal suspicion that obesity must be the visible sign of a poor or weak character. Rarely does anyone state this view so bluntly, but they don't have to. A cultural prejudice against overweight people says it silently and with a devastating effect on its victims. Think of the word FAT. What kind of associations do you have?

This prejudice against people who are fat is possibly the single greatest cause of self-hatred in our culture. It is a self-hatred that breeds an endless variety of other emotional disorders and that feeds a multi-billion dollar industry dedicated to providing salves and quick-but-false solutions to tens of millions of unhappy people. It is a self-hatred that is wholly undeserved.

From experimental data, scientists studying the causes of obesity have developed a few theories, a few conclusions, and many unanswered questions. One thing is clear: people who are statistically overweight are no more or less guilty of poor or weak character than anyone else. Some are simply big people: men and women who are born programmed to develop large fat deposits and who therefore are naturally heavy. Others have a tendency to store energy as fat when they fail to match their food intake to their energy needs; as a result, they experience major increases in weight. This is in contrast to people who maintain a consistent weight, who also eat more than they need, but whose bodies use other means to dispose of the excess.

A tendency toward being overweight and being obese might be regarded as an illness or disability only to the extent that it impairs health and shortens life: a circumstance that is rarer than is generally supposed. **Most large-scale studies of the relationship between health, longevity, and weight have shown that heavy people live as long as average weight people. In fact, underweight has been shown to be far more hazardous than overweight.** Because fat people are at risk for **different** illnesses than thin people are, it is often assumed (even by medical professionals) that obesity is associated with sickness.

Unfortunately, many healthy but large people are less concerned about their lifespan than about the impact of their size and shape on their social life and self-esteem. Too often their reaction to the unremitting discrimination they experience is to seek cosmetic changes in their appearance through endless varieties of malnutrition that they prefer to think of as "dieting."

Paradoxically and tragically, for many people the net effect of their attempts to lose weight is to further aggravate the tendency their bodies have to store fat. Worse, in the process they often sharpen their appetites, making their excess eating even more lively. It is these side effects of dieting and being overweight that we are principally concerned with in this book—side effects that have immense social, psychological, and physical consequences for people who suffer from them. They constitute a syndrome of disorders that includes anorexia, bulimia, bulimarexia, and compulsive eating.

All these aberrations have the distressing effect of alienating people from one of life's chief pleasures—eating—and of making an enemy of a healthy natural attribute—appetite. It has become customary to refer to them as **eating disorders,** and they are clearly that. At a more fundamental level, however, the struggle is with

Physicians divide obesity into endogenous and exogenous. Endogenous means something wrong with the body like an underactive thyroid gland. Exogenous means eating too much. Many physicians label fat people "exogenous obesity" to represent their belief that fatness is from gluttony.

appetite. It is not the act of eating that has become disordered but the **urge** to eat that cannot be properly regulated. This gives rise to the extreme behaviors of self-starvation on the one hand and outrageous bingeing on the other. The bingeing, in turn, may instigate compensatory measures such as deliberate vomiting or purging.

For these reasons, we have coined the term *pathorexia,* meaning "disordered appetite," to refer to the whole spectrum of appetite and eating disorders. Pathorexia is a general term that incorporates anorexia, bulimia, bulimarexia, and other psychosomatic disorders of eating and appetite. It is not the first general term that has been used in this connection. In the 1960s, the word *dysorexia* was proposed, and later *dietary chaos syndrome* was used.

What we want to convey by using a general term such as pathorexia is the close relationship and interchangeability frequently seen among eating disorders. Some therapists and treatment centers have adopted the term pathorexia, but it is not widely used. More often the older but less accurate term *eating disorder* is used. Lately, the general phrase, *problems with food,* has found some currency.

A helpful concept for forming an understanding of pathorexia comes from considering the difference between appetite and hunger. **Appetite** describes an emotional and physical impulse to eat, regardless of nutritional needs. In contrast, **hunger** refers to a physical urge to eat caused by an immediate dietary deficiency.

In healthy people, hunger and appetite usually coincide. The occasions when they do not coincide include opportunities to eat treats and exotic offerings that arouse appetite even when we are not hungry. On the other hand, traumatic events can be so unsettling that appetite is lost even though hunger pain and the need for food are present.

When appetite disorders, or pathorexia, develop, the relationship between the desire to eat and the body's need for food is so discrepant that normal, healthy eating becomes the exception rather than the rule. This book is about those discrepancies, their causes, and their relationship to dieting, to being overweight, and to obesity. It is also a guide to their prevention and cure.

There is a distinct and crucial difference between pathorexic persons and fat persons who do not overeat but who are simply naturally heavy. The range of naturally healthy human shapes is far greater than fashion dictates, and many (perhaps most) soft, round people are content with their lives, their appetites, and their bodies. They diet from time to time, and may talk about how much they would like to lose weight, but their good common sense prevents them from going to harmful extremes.

In Chapter 3, we deal specifically with problems related to obesity. Chapter 10 includes some psychologically safe programs that can be used for weight loss. But we are primarily addressing **eating** and **appetite** disorders, not weight itself. The principal goal of this book is to help you distinguish between problems of eating, appetite, and weight, and to understand how they relate to each other.

Much of what has been written on eating disorders has concentrated on the life-threatening extreme of *anorexia nervosa*. We will not ignore this disturbing illness, but both our clinical work and this book deal mostly with the concerns of people whose appetite disorders, though painful and handicapping, are not so severe as to separate them from their families and friends. We want to promote understanding and provide relief for those millions of people whose struggle with physical, familiar, and social pressures has caused them to lose touch with their appetites and has set them in conflict with their own bodies.

SUMMARY

We live in a world that prizes slenderness and often condemns fatness, even though above average weight and even extreme fatness need not be a health hazard. There are widespread social and medical prejudices against heavy people. This gives rise to much self-hatred among fat people and causes a fear of fat among average and lightweight people. Fear of fat then influences these individuals to attempt weight loss at almost any expense. Fear of fat is a thread that runs repeatedly through this text. It is a fear that can undermine good physical and emotional health, a fear that can compel healthy young people to become entangled in a life-threatening web of eating disorders.

CHAPTER REVIEW

◆ ─────────VOCABULARY───────── ◆

appetite an emotional and physical desire to consume something. In the case of food, one may have an appetite regardless of nutritional needs.

compensatory Making up for something (bragging when insecure; forcing vomiting after a binge).

hunger physical urge to eat that is prompted by immediate need for energy.

pathorexia disordered appetite. Refers to the whole spectrum of food disorder problems.

purging forced cleansing or release. With eating disorders, usually by vomiting or laxative abuse.

◆ ─────FOR YOUR CONSIDERATION───── ◆

◆ Experiments with preschool children shown pictures of potential playmates found they chose thin and handicapped children over fat children. Why do you think this was so? Would it happen in other countries?

◆ At what age did you first learn of peers who dieted? What influence, if any, did this have on your behavior?

◆ The medical profession today is expected to perform many functions that are not associated with treating sickness. List examples where doctors treat and prescribe drugs for people who are not ill? How do you feel about the medical profession's responses to people who seek help to become more attractive or fashionable?

◆ When we are discouraged or disappointed many of us turn the problem inward and think things like: "If only I wasn't so tall, people would like me better," or, "If we lived in their neighborhood, they wouldn't ignore us." What do you think about "inner messages" like these? How do you think society influences these messages?

FROM DIET TO DISASTER
Varieties of Appetite Disorders

This chapter will help you:

1. Define six forms of pathorexia.

2. Understand the relationship of one appetite or eating disorder to another.

◆

"I get so embarrassed about eating that when I do it, it feels like I'm having sex in public."

We have identified six ways in which people experience appetite or eating disorders or pathorexia. They are: simple overeating, simple anorexia, anorexia nervosa, bulimia, bulimarexia, and oral expulsion. In this chapter we discuss each of these disorders individually. At the end there is a questionnaire that can be used to help rate the degree of pathorexia.

Experts disagree about the names and definitions used to describe appetite disorders. Some prefer to regard all appetite disorders as varieties of anorexia nervosa. Others do not distinguish between bulimia and bulimarexia. Some writers refer to "anorexic-like behavior," the "binge and purge syndrome," and "bulimia nervosa." There is even less agreement about what overeating is. Using the term pathorexia is our way of simplifying the matter. All these other terms are varieties of pathorexia.

SIMPLE OVEREATING

"Every time something goes wrong I want to eat, and every time something goes right I want to eat! When am I ever going to stop eating?"

Simple overeating is by far the commonest form of eating disorder. It is the way people respond to the loss of their natural ability to match their food intake with their energy output. For overeaters, the desire to eat almost always exceeds their need for food, so they either diet in an attempt to lose weight or they allow their appetite free rein and store excess calories as fat.

We explain in Chapters 6 and 7 how a variety of physical and psychological factors operate to encourage eating and inhibit restraint, making overeaters extra sensitive to some environmental cues that trigger eating.

Because our culture abounds in cues inviting us to eat, many overeaters are able to avoid excess intake only by adopting special controls, such as diets, calorie counting, or behavior modification programs, that temporarily enable them to cut out what tempts them. Some only find "success" with stapled stomachs, gastric bubbles, or wired jaws.

A woman in her early 40s who had always been classified as obese told us of a life made miserable by her weakness for eating. She began every day with a resolution to eat only three balanced meals, but she rarely got beyond 10 o'clock in the morning without being seduced by something tasty. By evening, all semblance of her resolve was gone, and she would make a stop at the refrigerator or the pantry each time she moved around the house.

Overeaters resist focusing their attention on their appetite, even though they are well aware of the problems it creates for them.

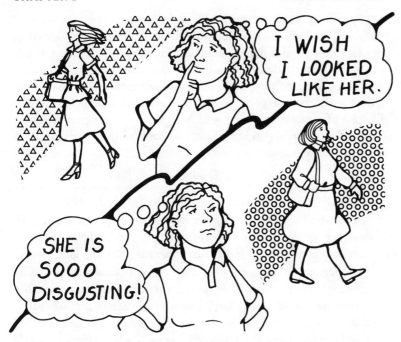

Figure 2-1. *Simple overeaters rank us all.*

They worry instead about their bodies, which they see as disfigured with excess fat. They look constantly for a simple and easy cure that will cause fat to melt away.

Most overeaters experiment with appetite suppressing medications of some kind, either over-the-counter or prescription. Although by doing so they acknowledge that it is their urge to eat that is the problem, they rarely grasp the full importance of that concept. Instead, they think only of losing weight and view the pills as a means to that end, not as a way to experience living without the desire to overeat.

Simple overeaters are usually very unhappy about their behavior patterns but mask their feelings with a facade of good humor. They often make jokes about their weight or the way they eat. Underneath, however, they worry chronically about their appearance. Some overeaters monitor every person they meet, every person they even catch sight of, and rank them all on a scale of thin to fat (Figure 2-1). In this way they keep track of their own place in a dismal and phony hierarchy. They envy the thin and despise the obese in an emotional tug of war that never offers them balance and harmony.

Overeaters adopt many tricks to help them deny or conceal their weight and their undisciplined eating. But every device of dress or posture and every public display of self-denial that is followed by secret eating serves to increase their sense of isolation and chips away at their self-esteem. Sharing their weakness with fellow sufferers is a great tension reliever, so groups like TOPS (Take Off Pounds Sensibly) and Weight Watchers provide them with valuable boosts in self-respect so long as they are willing to diet as a rite of passage for group membership.

Jessica

At 15, Jessica cried daily over her "too fat" body. Her mom was worried about this weight problem, too, since she had herself been a chubby teenager. When Jessica pleaded for help, her mom was only too happy to support treatment through the local weight loss program. Wise mom, ever aware of how hard it is to keep off weight once lost, did add her own motivational technique: If Jessica gained back more than a tiny percentage of any weight lost, she would owe her mother for the total cost of the weight loss program. Little did either of them realize that this contract would soon establish Jessica as a full-fledged bulimic.

SIMPLE ANOREXIA

"Really, I'd rather DIE than gain a single pound! I mean it! I mean it!"

Simple anorexia is a severe and unhealthy restriction of eating. Even though victims experience no loss of appetite, they reject most opportunities to eat, and lose as much as one-fifth of their normal weight. Most simple anorexics appear to be on the verge of starvation; but some, whose normal figures are a bit rounded, manage to look very fashionable.

An anorexic wrote in her diary for us: "I'm trying to figure out in calories what I had today—I look pregnant! This morning, coffee and melon = 50. Lunch, salad and lo-cal dressing = 50. Supper, salad and lo-cal dressing = 50, piece of flounder = 70, 1/3 cup green beans = 30, one roll = 70, package jello = 32. Total = 342 calories. It could be worse, I suppose."

Even though their stated reason for losing weight is cosmetic, anorexics who look physically too frail to be attractive, with hollow cheeks, thinning hair, and dark circles under their eyes, remain determined not to regain weight. They cannot see themselves as thin. Intensely afraid of being overweight and obese, they prefer to be skeletal rather than soft-textured and regard even their vestigial fat (minute remaining amounts of fat) with distaste.

While often feeling faint and suffering other symptoms of malnutrition, anorexics are surprisingly resilient and cope effectively with most aspects of everyday life.

Anna (Read)

Anna weighed 78 pounds when we met her for the first time. At five feet two inches, she seemed desperately gaunt to us. Nevertheless, she was maintaining a full schedule of high school activities, doing well academically, and keeping a place on the cheerleading squad. When she passed out at a practice one afternoon, the coach urged her to get a physical examination, but Anna rallied and talked her way out of taking action.

Only when she passed out for the third time was she taken to the school nurse. Anna resisted every attempt to get her into treatment until she was forced to choose between seeing a therapist or being dropped as a cheerleader.

Many anorexics impose extra burdens upon themselves. They undertake rigorous regimens of running, swimming, situps, or dancing—not to improve physical fitness, but in pursuit of further weight loss. They survive for the duration of the disease—often many years—on diets that appear to defy the basic principles of sound nutrition.

Anorexics are generally resistant to the most earnest and sincere efforts of their families and therapists to get them to eat reasonable meals or to set weight goals for them to work toward. This defiance has led many observers to conclude that family conflicts provoke much anorexic behavior. Indeed, family counseling often helps parents, brothers, and sisters avoid attitudes that promote or reinforce the self-starvation.

The very urgings of others toward improved eating may intensify the anorexic's symptoms. After all, a **need for control** is the foundation of severe food restriction. Continuing to diet strictly is a method of exerting control over those who would seek to change the anorexic.

But it is clear, too, that many anorexics are primarily interested in pursuing thinness because they are convinced it improves their appearance. And they get plenty of support for this view. People compliment them on how well they wear clothes; they have no trouble getting dates; friends and acquaintances envy their slimness and self-discipline.

Anorexia, which means "without appetite," may be a misnomer for this variety of pathorexia, for anorexics are often consumed with thoughts of food. They may spend hours preparing meals for other people and are almost always ready to get into discussions about restaurants or recipes. Typically, too, they indulge in binges from time to time, often eating large amounts of rather unappetizing food like bread, peanut butter, and cottage cheese, although simple carbohydrates remain their first choice.

They also hoard food in drawers and wardrobes, and then eat secretly, later throwing up what they have consumed. Their appetite, then, is more suppressed than lost, although after long periods without eating it may be much reduced.

There are indications that some anorexics may be responding to a minor brain dysfunction. This suggests the possibility that they may be physically predisposed to this disorder, and when they experience the stresses that come with adolescence, they instinctively begin to starve themselves.

Anorexia is often the first type of pathorexia to be observed in a patient. Because of the metabolic changes caused by the fasting and because eating remains a troubling behavior even after recovery, anorexics may subsequently develop other forms of appetite disorder.

Many anorexics know they are caught in a self-deluding web. Debbie, a high school sophomore, told us about hers.

·Debbie

"*Intellectually I didn't think that if I lost weight my problems would go away, but at another level I did. Every time I tricked my folks into thinking I'd had a meal but I hadn't, I felt strong and in control. It was the same when I weighed myself and I was lighter. . . . I stopped looking at the numbers after awhile, they scared me; all I cared about was that I was just a bit less each time.*"

Debbie described how at times she would become more realistic, but that caused trouble, too. "If I lost a whole pound I'd say to myself, 'This is ridiculous, you've got to stop this. You know what you're doing to yourself!' and I'd go have a snack. But it never ended there. I'd raid the refrigerator, then the pantry. Then I'd just keep eating because I'd know I was going to throw up. It was awful."

Despite their handicap, anorexics are usually very courteous in social and—initially at least—therapeutic contacts. But the facade of being polite, calm, agreeable, and hardworking provides only a poor mechanism for dealing with anxiety, envy, disappointment, or aggression.

Anorexics are ill-equipped for adolescence and adulthood, where more competition, harsher skills, and thicker skins are required. Confused about meeting these challenges, they pull back from growing up, turn anger inward, and seek control of unwelcome emotions through self-starvation. "I was so angry I could have lost 20 pounds!" expresses a common sentiment.

Such passive-aggressive behavior confounds their parents, about whom anorexics feel more intensely ambivalent than do normal adolescents.

Once the disorder has been identified, a battle royal may develop within the family, with parents pulled in many directions in their attempts to restore a traditional structure and order while their anorexic teenaged daughter typically explains that being left alone is all she needs.

By making her body the focus of conflict with her parents, a teenager gains immense power and influence. After all, for all practical purposes, only she can decide whether or not to eat. But the struggle is always more complex than the anorexic person anticipates. Family patterns of behavior do not change quickly, and the body has its own resources for counteracting the dangers of starvation. So the control an anorexic perceives in dieting is often lost when her appetite overcomes her willpower and a binge occurs.

Anorexic victims are at odds with society, using their bodies as weapons, but they find their bodies rebel against them, too. It is hard to imagine the loneliness they feel when this happens, but their typical response is to redouble the effort to conquer their appetites rather than accept defeat. They bitterly resist the need for adequate restoration, and they refuse to seek comfort and support from loved ones.

ANOREXIA NERVOSA

Anorexia nervosa is simple anorexia carried to the point of insanity. The woman quoted here was five feet tall and weighed 56 pounds when she argued with her therapist about her condition.

"Of course I'm still fat! Look at this, and this, and this! It's fat!"

In this state of self-starvation, the appetite is truly lost, and body weight is at least 15 percent below normal. Victims lose all sense of reality with regard to food intake and, believing that they have conquered the need to eat, may literally starve to death. This may be the most lethal of the psychiatric disorders. It is self-destructive and unquestionably a form of suicide.

Persons suffering from anorexia nervosa require hospitalization and intensive medical and psychiatric intervention. Even then they remain in grave danger.

Identifying the line that divides simple anorexia, which is best treated on an outpatient basis, from anorexia nervosa, which is

In the United States, psychiatric diagnoses are officially listed in a reference book called *The Diagnostic and Statistical Manual of Mental Disorders* (third edition, revised), or DSM-III-R for short. According to this source, only anorexia nervosa and bulimia nervosa are recognized as identifiable eating disorders. However, there is a catchall diagnosis called Other or Atypical Eating Disorders that allows mental health workers a lot of leeway in determining whether a patient is diagnosably sick. According to DSM-III-R:

- *Anorexia nervosa* is a refusal to maintain a body weight above 85 percent of anticipated weight for height and age, with an absence of corresponding physiological cause for low weight. Also required for a full diagnosis is amenorrhea (loss of periods), severe distortion of body image, and an intense fear of becoming obese.
- *Bulimia nervosa* is marked by uncontrollable episodes of bingeing, which may or may not be followed by a purge phase. Body weight is above 85 percent of expected weight. Again, an intense fear of obesity is observed.

There is still much controversy surrounding the diagnosis and naming of problems with food. We are not alone in using criteria that are absent from the official manuals. Our descriptors are derived from clinical experience with our own patients and from extensive consultations with other professionals in the field.

not, is a matter for careful professional judgment. Apart from substantial weight loss and associated physical problems, other considerations, such as the age of the patient, the degree of family discord, and the willingness to accept hospitalization, must be assessed. The younger the patient is, the more profoundly anorexic behavior may be seen as a cry for help—help to be rescued from the family, making at least a brief hospitalization the preferred treatment.

Severe anorexics almost invariably resent intrusion by family and physicians. They frequently attempt to hide their weight loss by wearing bulky clothing. When not closely supervised, they sometimes conceal heavy objects in their pockets or drink large quantities of water prior to being weighed. One patient forced a roll of coins up her vagina to falsely increase her weight.

When fed against their will, they often vomit their meals to prevent weight gain.

Chrissy

A *nurse used the term* **twilight zone** *to describe the tragedy of losing a patient in intensive care to starvation.*

"Chrissy was as nice a person as you could meet if you just wanted to talk. But as soon as nutrition in any form was proposed, she turned cold as ice. As far as she was concerned, we were assassinating her with our equipment, so she had a right to be angry. She said to me once, 'Starving keeps me sane.' "

Chrissy sabotaged every attempt that was made to get food into her. "The day before she died, she was so weak she could barely move, but she still managed to put a crimp in her intravenous tube to stop it working and then figured out how to disconnect the alarm. So it was an hour before we realized what she'd done. When we were cleaning her room afterward, we found two boxes of laxatives taped to the underside of the shelf in her cabinet."

Anorexia nervosa originally was seen primarily in wealthy, high-status families. Today, however, we see persons of all ages, both sexes, and every social class becoming caught up in weight phobia, punitive dieting, and appetite disorders, although young people from wealthy professional families may still predominate in clinic caseloads. And, according to recent research that links dieting behaviors among high school females to future eating disorders, these disorders will be with us a long time.

Severely impaired anorexics may suffer from a wide range of associated disabilities. They have a very poor understanding of their physical and emotional states. Body size and shape, for example, is a matter of great confusion for many, who believe they are far larger and fatter than they are. They often have lost the ability to recognize hunger or satiety. Sometimes this confusion extends to their emotions: patients may not know whether they are sad, angry, or even pleased, and may ask a parent or therapist to interpret their mood for them.

These distortions and deficits leave anorexics with little sense of control or trust. By focusing their entire attention on food, eating, exercise, and weight loss, they create the self-illusion of appropriate behavior while effectively isolating themselves from the corrective feedback and evaluations of their peers and family.

Left alone, they may become lethally turned in on themselves. Yet they have a terrible fear of having their insane world invaded. Only caring therapists and an awakened family can lead them back to the real world.

BULIMIA

"I stuff myself until my stomach hurts; but that just slows me down. I don't quit until the food's all gone."

Also known as **hyperphagia,** bulimia includes a variety of eating disorders all characterized by episodes of voracious eating. On these occasions, outrageous bingeing may be indulged, during which anything and everything edible is stuffed into the mouth. The binges often end only when all available food has been consumed or when the victim's stomach is so full that further eating becomes impossible. Some even binge to the point of passing out. While bingeing, bulimics often feel peacefully removed from reality. Afterward, they are likely to feel intense remorse, vowing to themselves that it will never happen again. But their promise is rarely kept for long. The major reason for bulimia is that victims simply give up the fight to control a seemingly insatiable desire to eat, and allow their appetite unrestrained expression.

> *Many of our clients could identify with the women who told us, "During the fat times in my life I had to force myself to go to work. Then I would rush home, pull the shades, unhook the phone, and sit on the floor next to the refrigerator, eating myself into a stupor."*

Typically, bulimics feel very guilty about their behavior, which causes them to be secretive about eating. In family settings, where secretive eating may be impossible, young bulimics may attempt to manipulate their parents into both curbing and permitting their overeating. An example of this was a child who requested that a lock be put on the refrigerator and that she be provided with a key!

Bulimics are just as anxious about weight and fat as other pathorexics, and their massive binges usually provoke substantial gains. The conflict between their craving to eat and the fear of obesity is often reduced by planning for binges, by fasting, or limiting intake to low-calorie snacks, tea, or diet soda for several days.

Many bulimics find that they can easily keep up a pattern of weekend indulgence preceded and followed by weekday frugality. Some binge only once a month, saving both money and calories, so their overeating, once begun, can be of monumental proportions.

In one common variety of bulimia, a small surprise or upset triggers the hyperphagia. A party, a holiday, a rejection by a friend, or some other negative experience will do. Outside influence can then be blamed for the loss of control that follows. At a deeper level of awareness, the bulimic person knows, of course, that sooner or later the opportunity for indulgence will occur and will be taken. Once the binge is under way, the excuse for beginning it is forgotten.

Often the search for food becomes an obsession. Sometimes civilized behavior is abandoned if the only way to get food is through threats or theft.

"*One evening when I was totally out of control and there was nothing in the house, I raided garbage cans outside the apartments. I sorted through stuff until I found a piece of watermelon and had started to eat it when a guy came by with a bag of garbage. He looked at me strangely, but he didn't know what I was doing, and when he'd gone, I just kept on eating. I kept on eating out there by the garbage cans as long as I found things to stuff in my mouth. It was after that night that I realized just how much I needed help.*"

Normal eaters also binge occasionally, and simple overeaters often report bingeing behaviors. Inquiry usually reveals that such episodes are relatively minor compared with the enormous intake of a true bulimic. A hyperphagic binge may consist of several pounds of food, perhaps as much or more than a family of four would consume in a day. Doughnuts by the dozen, ice cream by the carton, bread by the loaf, and peanut butter by the jar are the measure of quantity for the established bulimic.

Some studies describe the binge as highly individual. A person with a strong mental image of a need for **severe** food restriction, will consider as little as two cookies to be a binge. Such a person will suffer all the guilt and remorse that big volume bingers experience.

Older and wealthier bulimics sometimes regulate and excuse their disorder by eating out. It is easier to justify a binge if someone else has a hand in its preparation. In all-you-can-eat restaurants, such behavior can even be considered as having the endorsement of the management! There have been reports in the press of customers in these restaurants becoming so full they collapsed and died.

BULIMAREXIA

"At first I used to throw up to compensate for bingeing, but then I realized I was only bingeing so that I could throw up."

As its name implies, this disorder is a combination of bulimic and anorexic behaviors. Bingeing is followed by purging with laxatives or self-induced vomiting. The cycle of binge and purge may be regularly spaced—a week or so apart—or it may be sporadic and unpredictable. Some victims are driven to frequent minor binges, such as eating a box of cookies and then quickly throwing up. This latter behavior may be repeated as often as 20 times a day, taking the place of normal meals.

The term bulimarexia was coined by a psychologist at Cornell University, Marlene Boskind-White, who discovered that scores of women students were bingeing and purging. In her view, bulimarexia is a **learned** behavior that can be corrected by learning better behaviors, backed by healthier attitudes about oneself. We agree with her, but we think the problem is more complex than that. In our experience, many people with bulimarexic symptoms become enmeshed in physical and psychological complications resulting from the behavior that limit their freedom to give it up. They become hooked on the release of endorphin that is associated with purging, for example. For this reason, we believe that bulimarexia is not just a behavior. It is a disease.

Bulimarexia can be viewed as an extreme version of the simple overeater's pattern of excess eating followed by strict dieting. But anorexics and bulimics also drift into bulimarexic behavior. The discovery that purging or vomiting makes it easier to indulge a disordered appetite becomes an irresistible but guilt-inducing temptation. The secrecy and self-hatred that result cause victims to withdraw from their friends and family. They become so addicted to the behavior that they avoid social contacts so they can binge and purge unobserved. A bulimarexic woman talked about how she felt when she could not purge:

"It's amazing how tense I get. Last night we had the in-laws for dinner, and I couldn't get to the bathroom. I went to bed without purging because Craig was following me around. He said I ground my teeth in my sleep all night and kept him awake. In the morning he had to massage my neck for 10 minutes before I could move my head."

Bulimarexics can be distinguished from anorexics and bulimics by the emphasis they learn to place on vomiting or purging. Eating gradually comes to serve principally as an introduction to the main event: the expulsion or expurgation.

A 30-year-old executive described to us how she coped with the constant anxiety she felt about her daily round of business meetings. "I keep dozens of small packets of saltines in my desk, in my purse, and hidden all over the building. Right before I have to talk with someone, I stuff a few crackers down, slip into a bathroom and bring them up again. Somehow the routine helps me get through the day."

The Degrees of Abuse

Involvement in food abuse ranges from isolated incidents to full-scale addiction, as described in the following hierarchy:

Isolated: Disconnected episodes once or twice a year with little or no temptation to abuse between these times. Frequent nonabusive dieting and minor weight fluctuations may occur.

Occasional: Up to once-a-month episodes of food or laxative abuse with more frequent fantasies and temptations. This person may be plagued by a chronic concern about weight and want to diet.

Routine: Regularly occurring food abuse contingent on predictable events (e.g., throwing up after Sunday dinner with family). Chronic preoccupation with food and weight also is a symptom.

Habitual: An at least weekly pattern of food abuse, sustained by an unwillingness to make the effort to break out of a cycle that is clearly maladaptive and hazardous.

Obsessive: Daily involvement in abusive eating or fasting/purging behaviors that are the most important part in the daily routine and felt to be essential for functioning, yet known to be self-destructive.

Addictive: Daily pattern of abuse interferes with virtually all other aspects of life. The pattern is sustained mostly to ward off the pain of withdrawal, and to combat the fear of being without the symptoms that now lend structure to life.

Partial remission: With treatment, bulimics and anorexics are often able to give up habitual food abuse, although they may redevelop symptoms during times of stress.

Our experience with patients indicates that the appetite disorder becomes symbolic of emotions that are felt but cannot be directly expressed. People who long to be loved but feel rejected may turn to food for comfort. They then punish and cleanse themselves by purging, a gesture that symbolizes both anger toward themselves and against the people who reject them.

There are other needs met in the binge and purge cycle, the most frequently reported being a brief sense of well-being that follows the episode. Many bulimarexics see their symptoms as an opportunity to totally let go of all restraint, thus compensating themselves for their sense of being overcontrolled in the rest of their lives.

An anxious salesman told us how he relieves tension. "There are certain restaurants I have found that have bathrooms with an outer door I can lock. I go to these restaurants when I'm in the mood and really relax and enjoy the meal, knowing that I can get rid of the food fast, before I leave, and no one will be listening in the next stall."

Unfortunately, the behavior itself quickly becomes addictive. Instead of gaining control, bulimarexics lose further control of their lives. This may set the stage for a variety of emotional disorders, especially chronic depression.

There is a special type of pathorexia that afflicts some athletes and people who are professional dancers and fashion models. These people have a great deal of their sense of identity, well-being, and security invested in their physical prowess or appearance.

For such people, success depends on consistently winning under fierce competition. They have learned to be very disciplined with regard to training and diet in order to preserve their victor's edge. Sometimes athletes and dancers discover that they can improve their performance by starving off fat and lean tissue while maintaining their strength through strict workouts of the muscles they use most.

The lost weight allows them to improve their speed and stamina or qualifies them to compete against lighter competitors. But the starving also triggers their appetite, as their bodies strive to regain lost substance. This change in appetite is unexpected and unwelcome. These intensely competitive people find themselves in another struggle, one for which they are ill-prepared. The result may be an attack of bulimia, which usually changes to bulimarexia.

Athletes and dancers who seek help for their eating disorder think they are faced with choosing between giving up their addiction and thus lowering their performance and risking their careers, or remaining addicted. In our clinical experience, they view performance as too precious to be sacrificed, and accept pathorexia as the price of victory.

We were doing a call-in TV show one evening when a viewer identified herself as a member of the 1968 U.S. Olympic Gymnastic Team. She said that at that time she and everyone else on the squad was bulimic. All the girls, she said, had discovered they had steadier nerves after purging. She also said the coaches knew what was going on, but ignored it because they saw it improved performance.

The situation is similar for models. When they discover they can be more successful if they look more cadaverous, they accept semi-starvation as the cost of staying in business.

It is a very human trait to choose visible, short-term gains rather than heed the dangers of invisible, long-term risks. For many people, a few years of forced vomiting seems trivial when compared with success in competition or prominence and fame as a celebrity. Consider the example of Jane Fonda, who admits to 20 years of bulimia to maintain an acceptable figure for the movies.

It seems to us an awful irony that many men and women who are regarded as talented or beautiful and who serve as role models to others live in a state of semi-starvation and suffer the painful consequences of chronic malnutrition.

We do not know how long performers have endured pathorexia. Because secrecy has been the rule until recently, generations of people may have believed they were alone in this behavior. Or perhaps our 20th-century culture has created stresses that lead many people to adopt extreme measures that only a tiny minority felt driven to in the past.

Jeff

Jeff became bulimarexic with the help of his baseball coach. A good slugger, Jeff's liability was his slowness in running the bases. Each time Jeff was put out, his coach would make a point of speculating what the score might have been "if Jeff were 20 pounds livelier."

Then Jeff came down with a serious stomach virus that lasted two weeks and left him 10 pounds lighter. To everyone's surprise, Jeff was visibly faster in his first game back. Even his girlfriend complimented him on his sleeker appearance.

It was all Jeff needed. Through dieting, he lost another 10 pounds and started running on days when there were no games. Jeff, who had never before given a thought to what he ate, started watching every bite. He found that the pizza and beer suppers that followed almost every game, and that had once seemed as much fun as the game itself, were now occasions of inner conflict—until he learned to throw up as soon as he got home.

When Jeff sought treatment a few months later, he was vomiting after each meal. He had become obsessed with his baseball statistics, his figure, and his wardrobe. He had completely lost sight of his established identity as a carefree, husky hitter who left finesse and grooming to his less well-endowed friends.

ORAL EXPULSION SYNDROME

The oral expulsion syndrome (OES) occurs only occasionally. We believe a prominent entertainer was the first person to broadcast to the world the technique of losing weight by chewing food and spitting it out instead of swallowing it. We have found that a few people who experiment with this behavior become addicted to it. They spend hours doing it in secret and, in time, develop intense anxieties about swallowing. As a consequence, they become isolated, fearful, and seriously malnourished.

Not much is known about OES. We do not know how common it is, who does it, and how many people who try it become addicted. We can see aspects of every other form of pathorexia represented in the behavior. We have come to think of it as a low-key, low-profile pathorexia, the kind that a disciplined, cautious person might get caught up with. The following case study is a composite of some of the examples we have seen.

Gladys

Gladys developed OES at age 37, shortly after her husband left her for a younger and, Gladys presumed, thinner woman. She began dieting furiously with a determination that was fueled by her anger at being abandoned. Soon, however, she developed an aversion to swallowing. "I went from having to force myself to swallow to believing that if I swallowed I would choke," she told us.

Because she was no longer consuming anything, Gladys felt free to put whatever she fancied in her mouth. Within a few weeks, she was spending her free time chewing or looking for food to chew. As her neurosis intensified, she began to fear that even the fruit juices she involuntarily swallowed were contaminating her.

Anorexia, bulimia, and bulimarexia are physically and psychologically debilitating disorders. The ill effects of starvation, bingeing, laxative abuse, and vomiting vary from person to person. Upsets in body chemistry, potassium deficiency, tooth decay, sore throat, liver damage, rectal bleeding, heart dysfunction, and chronic fatigue are common.

Most female victims experience some loss of menstrual function if there is significant weight loss. The inherent malnutrition slows tissue replacement. Cuts and sores heal more slowly. Forced vomiters sometimes develop infected abrasions on their hands from involuntary bites incurred while gagging themselves with their fingers.

Psychologically, the effects are seen in the gradual breakdown of honesty and sincerity. This begins with lying and deceit to conceal binges and stealing and shoplifting to finance them. The growing sense of worthlessness may trigger sexual adventurism. But the most common behavioral change is withdrawal from social contacts and increased involvement with the cycle of overeating, purging, fasting, or excessive exercise.

Gradually, even everyday activities such as shopping or being seen in public may become difficult. The disabilities may snowball until the severely pathorexic person lives in a world clouded with depression and imprisoned with anxiety. At last, the lonely victim seeks professional help or is forced into treatment by despairing parents or a judge.

Although there are many, many cases in which these disastrous consequences have occurred, we should not lose sight of the fact that there are also people who have forms of pathorexia that, while they are potentially hazardous, do not appear to be especially handicapping. Some people with the medical disorder inflammatory bowel disease find temporary relief in forced vomiting. This can lead to episodes of eating and purging that mimic bulimia, but are quite unrelated to the psychiatric disorder. We have had brief consultations with many people who admit to a variety of appetite disorders but who claim that they feel fine. Some popular weight loss programs appear to be barely concealed forms of anorexia, bulimia, and bulimarexia.

SUMMARY

In 1983, the popular singer Karen Carpenter died from heart failure that was reportedly caused by a combination of starvation and laxative abuse. Others have reported that her death followed the use of ipecac. In any event, her death occurred at a time when she had regained a good deal of weight and was thought to be well on the road to recovery.

We believe these people are living dangerously. We know they are closing their eyes to reality. But we know, too, that their personal experience with pathorexia has been more positive than negative. In the eyes of the victim, the reward of thinness is worth risking any negative side effects.

Some eventually abandon the behavior after a few weeks or after many years. Some hear about the dangers from other people and then seek treatment. Karen Carpenter's death caused many people to get help they never before believed they needed. We hope this book will be the trigger for change for some of our readers, and for the patients other readers will treat.

We use the accompanying questionnaire (pp. 32-33) to screen patients. You can use it to rate yourself. Note that the scoring is not quite as straightforward as you might suppose. In many questions the answer *seldom* is rated as healthier than *never*. This is because everyone experiences some appetite upset, and denying oneself completely is less healthy than living with a normal weakness.

CHAPTER REVIEW

◆ ———————————VOCABULARY——————————— ◆

amenorreah loss of the menstrual cycle.

anorexia nervosa self-starvation with at least 25 percent of original body weight lost. Victims also have amenorreah, fat phobia, and a severe distortion of body image.

bulimarexia bingeing followed by purging through laxative abuse, forced vomiting, or enema abuse.

bulimia uncontrolled eating in the presence of a strong desire to lose weight.

endorphin a painkilling chemical secreted by the body, with a structure and function similar to morphine.

ipecac nonprescription drug often recommended by pediatricians to be taken as an antidote for accidental poisoning.

oral expulsion syndrome (OES) chewing but never swallowing food. OES is a diet technique in some, but the reflection of emotional disturbance and eating disorder in most.

phobia unrealistic fear, often obsessional.

potassium an electrolyte or ion that is an **essential** mineral in the body's workings. When potassium is lacking, the nervous system cannot conduct messages properly.

simple anorexia severe and unhealthy restriction of food for fear of being fat. Anorexics have a severely distorted body image.

simple overeating the desire to eat beyond the need for food. Simple overeaters are chronically on diets and worried about their appearance.

◆ ———————FOR YOUR CONSIDERATION——————— ◆

◆ Problems with food are regrettably common. Without violating anyone's privacy, describe some problems you have observed. Do they fit the disorders you have read about here? Rank their severity using the "Degrees of Abuse" section on page 25.

◆ What are the characteristics of a healthy appetite? Describe a person you know who has no problems with food.

APPETITE DISORDERS QUESTIONNAIRE

Circle the answer that best describes you:

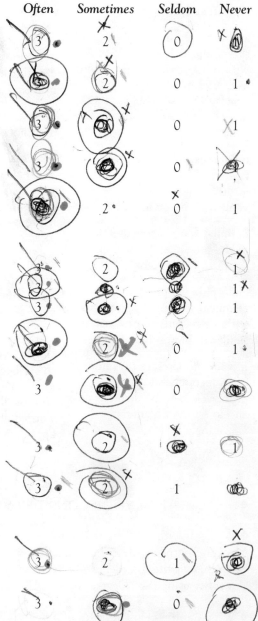

	Often	Sometimes	Seldom	Never
1. Do you have eating patterns that you suspect might be abnormal?	3	2	0	0
2. How frequently do you eat when you are not hungry?		2	0	1
3. Do you go for long periods without food when busy with other things?	3		0	1
4. Have you made unsuccessful attempts to lose weight by dieting?	3		0	
5. Are you especially attracted to breads and sweets?		2	0	1
6. Do you suspect that you are especially susceptible to the following aspects of food?				
smell	3	2		1
sight		2		1
thought of food	3	2		1
7. How frequently do you eat far more than your body needs before you feel full?		2	0	1
8. Do you feel uneasy if you cannot reach for a snack or drink between meals?	3		0	
9. Can you easily fall into long conversations about recipes, diets, restaurants, and other food-related topics?	3	2		1
10. Do you feel tormented by your love/hate feelings about eating?	3	2	1	
11. Have you ever maintained an abnormally low weight through strictly disciplined eating because you were afraid you would lose control if you tried to eat normally?	3	2	1	
12. Do you avoid eating in public and then eat secretly, shortly afterwards?	3		0	

APPETITE DISORDERS QUESTIONNAIRE

	Often	Sometimes	Seldom	Never
13. Can other people easily influence you to eat even when you are still digesting a good meal?			0	1
14. Do you reach for food to tranquilize you and then feel remorseful after you have eaten?	3		0	1
15. Have you secretly binged out of control in the past year?	3		0	1
16. Have you followed a binge with:				
induced vomiting or purging with laxatives or enemas?	6	4	3	
punitive fasting?	3	2	1	
17. Do you exercise to compensate for food you have eaten or plan to eat?	3			1

18. How many close blood relations (siblings, parents, aunts, uncles, grandparents) have been diagnosed as alcoholic, diabetic, hypoglycemic, or drug dependent?	**Over 6**	**3-5**	**1-2**	
	3	2	1	0

total points _____

2+0+3+2+3+2+0+2+1+0+2+0+2+0+0

65
0
+3
+1

38

2+2

Scoring and Interpretation

0—20 points:	Healthy appetite
21—30 points:	Hazardous appetite
31—40 points:	Moderately disordered appetite
41—66 points:	Severely disordered appetite

23

Use this questionnaire to clarify appetite and eating problems. Notice that occasional indulgence is more normal than rigid compliance with healthy behavior. The scoring is based on clinical studies but is intended to be suggestive, not definitive. This is not a diagnostic test.

OVERWEIGHT AND OBESITY
What It Really Means to be Heavy

This chapter will help you:

1. List various definitions of obesity.
2. Describe popular views of obesity.
3. Discuss the complexities of what causes obesity.
4. Evaluate the controversy around the consequences of obesity.

◆

*"From my point of view,
being fat has always meant
having to say you're
sorry."*

This chapter provides an overview of obesity and includes definitions and descriptions of popularly accepted views of the obese state. We also discuss conditions that may play a role in the causes of obesity. We conclude with a review of the consequences of obesity.

Throughout history, the female body has been an object of admiration and desire and the frequent subject of artists, poets, and writers. Works of some of the great masters—Michelangelo's angels in the Sistine Chapel, Renoir's bathers, the nymphs of Greek mythology, and the Venus de Milo—portray women with robust, full figures.

These works of art show beauty that is sensual, sensitive, compelling, and timeless. Yet many Western women would not express satisfaction with the Venus de Milo's measurements of 37-26-38. Instead, they strive for the "perfect" 36-24-36 form or even the "delightful" 31-24-33 measurements of the model Twiggy, who created a sensation in the 1960s with her unprecedented slenderness.

This quest for thinness, this desire to be light, is not universal. Obese women have also been highly sought after in many cultures at various periods of history. Some African tribes lock their pubescent females in fattening huts where they are denied exercise and receive extra rations of food for as long as two years. This practice produces an overweight woman who symbolizes the well-to-do status of her family.

Other cultures and connoisseurs discriminate in their preference for the location of fat deposits. Steatopygia (large buttocks and heavy upper thighs), a well-endowed bosom, or both combined with a small waist are classically fashionable choices for the female shape.

The pursuit of these proportions has led women to try a variety of devices and to submit to mutilations in an attempt to alter their natural physique. Although corsets and waist cinches caused fainting, rib fractures, and permanent distortions of the respiratory system, they remained in vogue for generations and can still be seen today in the costume of the Playboy bunny. Around the turn of the century, some women were reputed to have had ribs removed to achieve this shape.

More recently, silicone injections and breast implants have replaced the padded bra and bustle, revealing again an unceasing determination to conform to current ideals. A recent phase in this area involves breast reduction surgery and fat suctioning. The French are even reported to have a pill that induces the brain to release serotonin, the chemical that creates a feeling of satisfaction following the ingestion of carbohydrates. We fear that this will make becoming an anorexic even easier!

Obviously, although admiration for the female figure is universal, it is subject to much aesthetic interpretation. What is praised at a given place at a given time will be sought after by those women who do not naturally possess the currently "perfect" shape.

DEFINING OBESITY

Clinical interpretations of obesity are as varied as are cultural norms about what is attractive. Described below are some serious and not so serious methods for judging girth. Throughout this book, we repeatedly emphasize our concern that beliefs of what is overweight and obese must be determined individually by focusing on heredity and health. The material that follows demonstrates the controversy that exists in defining obesity.

One common method of determining the relationship between ideal weight and height for women is to allow yourself 100 pounds for the first 5 feet plus 5 pounds for each additional inch. A similar formula also states that if you subtract your waist measurement from your height and the result is less than 36 inches, you have a weight problem. A third equally general method says that you are overweight if, when lying on your back on a hard, flat surface, your stomach prevents a ruler from being placed from your breast bone to your pelvis (Figure 3-1). At one time, television commercials told us that if we could "pinch an inch" it was time to buy a certain sponsor's cereal.

These methods seem naive when held up to scientific scrutiny, and they have little relationship to beauty. We certainly know that some people are very healthy **and** very attractive at a variety of weights. In one of the above methods, a slight curve in the spine would allow for a great deal of weight to be put on the hips before a state of overweight would show up. None of the aforementioned methods takes musculature or age into account, and all reflect only the crudest of aesthetic values. To use such simplistic formulas to determine proper weight is foolish and potentially hazardous.

Scientific attempts to specify criteria for obesity have been equally varied, but typically have focused on the percentage of body weight made up of fat deposits.

This percentage has been determined with instruments that measure skinfold thicknesses around the body—a grownup version of the pinch an inch technique—and by using mathematical formulas that include body weight in air, body weight in water, and body volume. There are also sophisticated electronic and surgical

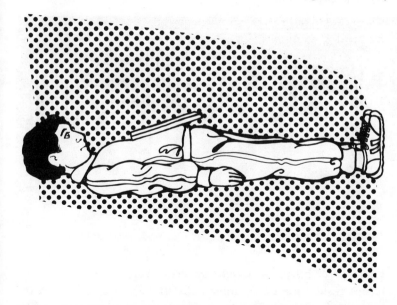

Figure 3-1. *Confirmation of overweight according to one popular method.*

techniques that calculate very precisely the ratio of fat to lean tissue. Some of these ratios are now derived by computers, although the method has not yet been validated.

In 1959, the Metropolitan Life Insurance Company published a chart of ideal weights that was the first one commonly used by health professionals. The tables offered a range of weights for various heights that people could interpret, based on their own understanding of their body structure. It was widely, but wrongly, believed that these charts provided an accurate measure of how much a person should weigh for optimal health. In fact, the figures averaged about 15 percent below the mean average weight of most healthy Americans, and the statistics were used to accuse millions of people of imprudent indulgence.

In 1983, new tables were published that contradicted the old charts and endorsed an upward expansion of the range for normal weight. Even though the new charts are better, they are still based on a population of insurance customers. They do not take age into account, and they are certainly not applicable to all individuals. We believe they are still too vague and biased to be especially useful. Further questions have also been raised about the influence of smoking on weight and longevity.

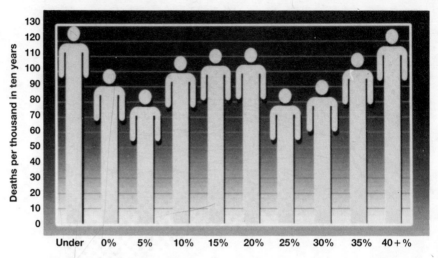

Figure 3-2. *Effects of weight on death rates. These data represent results from five major U.S. studies. The values on the horizontal axis represent the percent over the insurance tables "desirable" weight. For example, death rates for individuals at the "desirable" weight was 100; for persons 30% over the "desirable" weight, it was 91.*

Many large research studies with thousands of subjects in the United States and throughout the world who were observed for more than 20 years have failed to resolve questions about the relationships between health and weight (Figure 3-2). In most studies, associations between mortality and weight are quite small. Some find adiposity (fatness) to be an advantage, others show it to be a liability. One study of Harvard University graduates who were followed for 25 years showed that slow weight gainers survived better than men who remained at a steady weight. But no scientists have yet reported incontrovertible findings, so the debate continues.

These epidemiological studies have shown that only a minority of Americans conform to the Metropolitan Life ideals. The mean weight for adult American men and women of average height is about 20 percent above the recommendations. The average man stands 5 feet 9 inches tall and weighs 172 pounds, and the average women is 5 feet 4 inches tall and weighs 143 pounds. We know from census data that these people, especially the women, are likely to live longer than any Americans before them.

A sad and worrisome addition to these statistics comes from another Harvard study, which reported that 50 percent of American youth are much heavier and in poorer physical condition than their peers of only a decade before. Since heredity cannot account for this change, lifestyle must. It is especially sad that young people are getting off to such a poor start while older Americans are making great strides in reducing heart disease through healthier living.

Is weighing well above "average" unhealthy? For decades, physicians have admonished their adipose patients to reduce and then watched helplessly as those patients cycled through periods of loss followed by greater gain. Do such cycles occur because bad habits are impossible to overcome, or because the treatment is worse than the disease, or a little of both?

We believe it is vitally important to evaluate **why** a person is heavy. Large people with big bones are born to carry a lot of weight. These people may become underweight if they diet down to the national average or to Metropolitan Life norms. Others, who through ignorance or poor judgment adopt hazardous lifestyles with little physical activity and poor or excessive eating patterns, may develop obesity, which should be treated with changes in living. Still others may be fat **because** they diet repeatedly, and have ended with more gained than lost. Such people need to stop concentrating on their weight and learn how to moderate their eating behavior.

Because we think it is nonsense to burden people with the label obese unless their health is potentially in danger, we use a 30-percent cutoff as an initial measure of obesity. Figure 3-3 on the following page shows average weights for heights that were derived by combining data from a number of sources. These figures represent our own rough guide to minimal obesity, which is 30 percent over those means.

A recent study of adopted children in Denmark again confirmed that being overweight is predominantly determined by genetics. Labels such as obese may have little utility for health improvement when the "obesity" has been inherited.

It is important to recognize that the criterion for obesity used in Figure 3-3 is at best imprecise. We are using weight to indicate fatness, and that relationship is only approximate. Persons with substantial muscular development may be heavy without being obese, whereas others can be obese at lower weights. And in either case, obesity is not necessarily a liability.

IS BEING OVERWEIGHT UNHEALTHY?

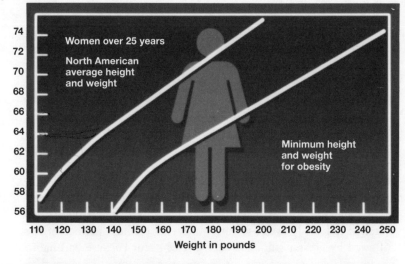

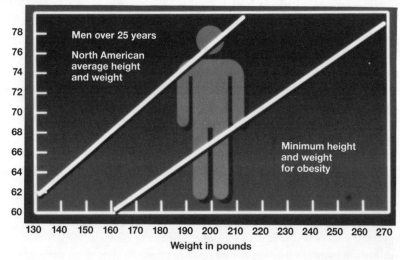

Figure 3-3. *Derived weights for heights based on selected national surveys.*

We repeat that there are no simple measures of obesity. It is essential to assess each case individually to decide whether a person has a health risk because of being overweight.

Note, too, that the obese weight for men and women of the same height differs by as much as 10 pounds. This is because the percentage of women's body weight that should be fat is roughly double the amount for men. Although there is much variation and overlap in this statistic, it is reasonable to expect healthy women to be softer and rounder than men.

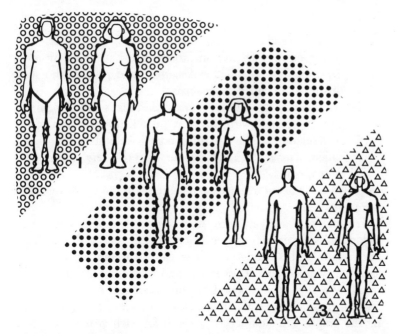

Figure 3-4. *Three major body types:* **1.** *A tendency to be soft and round and have substantial fat deposits. This is called* endomorphy, *and people who are high in this trait are called* endomorphs. **2.** *A tendency to be heavily muscled. This is called* mesomorphy, *and people high in this trait are called* mesomorphs. **3.** *A tendency to have a thin, bony, skeletal body. This is called* ectomorphy, *and people like this are called* ectomorphs.

Today's fashions seek to deny this natural trait, and the figures in Figure 3-3 are vastly different from what is generally considered attractive. It is a real and widespread tragedy that so many people are unable to accept their perfectly healthy bodies simply because they conform to biology and not to *Vogue* magazine.

Finally, we need to consider one other factor that is generally ignored: the effect of age on weight. Research studies confirm the belief that as people become middle-aged, many of them gain weight. This is not a universal phenomenon, however, and therein lies the problem that causes so much pain. Thoughtless people, both lay and professional, argue that because some persons retain an adolescent shape all their lives, everyone should stay thin.

This simplistic attitude ignores the immense differences in personality and physique that bring so much variety to our culture.

In Chapter 6 we explain in some detail that the human body can be categorized according to three major characteristics (Figure 3-4) that are inherited from parents and are not subject to change.

Each of us is a blend of all three characteristics, which are:

1. A tendency to be soft and round and have substantial fat deposits. This is called *endomorphy*, and people who show this trait are called *endomorphs*.
2. A tendency to be heavily muscled. This is called *mesomorphy*, and people with this trait are called *mesomorphs*.
3. A tendency to have a thin, bony, skeletal body. This is called *ectomorphy*, and people like this are called *ectomorphs*.

People who are about average on all three of these traits are called *midrangers*.

The effects of age vary with the type of body a person possesses. Endomorphs experience the most change; ectomorphs, the least. The nature of this change is a slow gain in weight up to around age 35 in women and 50 in men, then a leveling-off period, followed by a slow losing period beginning around 60 years of age. Because these changes affect the mean averages, young adults using the graphs can subtract 1.5 pounds for each year under 25 to get a closer approximation of their mean weight for their height.

Many environmental and psychological variables interfere with this process, with changes in diet and activity levels being the most significant. Endomorphic people clearly tend toward obesity, especially in middle age. Acknowledging that special liability and acting to minimize health hazards rather than pursuing unrealistic aesthetic goals can make enormous differences in their sense of well-being.

THE CAUSES OF OBESITY

"I know what causes obesity —it's everything I ever did or ever was!"

Established obesity is an almost irreversible condition, but our culture places such a high value on slimness that millions of Americans spend their lives struggling fruitlessly to be thin.

Obesity is a complex phenomenon that is still not fully understood by scientists, although the literature is rich with research attempting to isolate the causes. With the exception of the five percent of the cases that are attributable to physical dysfunction and hereditary diseases, there are no apparent causes for obesity. Research has revealed the significance of certain potentially key factors in understanding some obese populations. These factors are reviewed below.

Cell Growth During Infancy, Adolescence, and Pregnancy

As we discuss in more detail in Chapter 4, a major discovery of the late 1960s that was confirmed in the early 1970s was that fat cells are developed at certain critical periods of human growth. In infancy and adolescence, the body's inherited potential for fat cell development is mobilized, and **adipose tissue** (a fancy name for

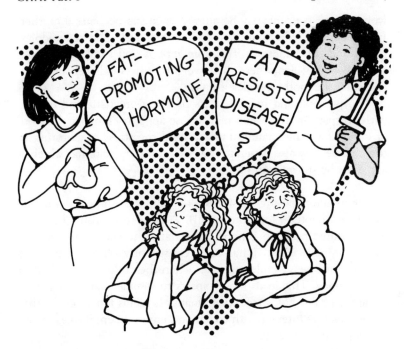

Figure 3-5. *The influences of pregnancy on weight gain.*

fat) is made. The amount of this growth depends on nutritional and environmental factors. These factors may cause the genetic potential to be unfulfilled or overdeveloped, according to individual circumstances.

Fat cells also develop during pregnancy, and more may appear when existing ones grow to their maximum size. Whenever this occurs, it creates a permanent addition to the body's tissue. Fat cells can shrink, but they do not disappear.

Studies indicate that for some women there is a relationship between pregnancy and the development of adult-onset obesity, but the cause of this phenomenon is not immediately clear.

Perhaps fat is developed by pregnant women because of the presence of fat-promoting hormones in their bodies that are needed by the fetus (Figure 3-5). Or pregnancy itself could permanently alter the need for and use of food. It is also possible that nature tries to endow mothers with more fat so they will be able to survive infectious diseases and care for their children.

Environmental changes may be responsible. Many women with infants and small children find it necessary to be in and around the home, they have less time to exercise, and they spend more time closer to and tempted by food. Another possibility is that a woman's self-concept may be altered once she becomes a mother. If this change reflects an abandonment of lithe and sexy adolescence and the adoption of a more serious and stable figure that suits becoming a mother, then weight gain could well be influenced by the motherhood self-image.

The physical and mental stress of being pregnant and dealing with postpartum depression may arouse appetite. Finally, the work of caring for a new family member and the stress of adjusting to the change may also generate the need for extra stamina, which is achieved by storing extra fat.

Hereditary Predisposition

Another factor causing obesity is a hereditary predisposition to fatness (see Chapter 4 for more detail). A clear relationship has been demonstrated between genetic factors and the occurrence of obesity in animals. And it has been consistently observed that big parents have heavy children, even when the children are raised in foster homes. This leads most experts to assume that what is true for animals also holds true for humans. It seems fair to claim that genetic factors interact with social and environmental ones in the development of obesity.

Possible Emotional Factors

Because we are all familiar with the natural human tendency to seek simple comforts like food when we are troubled, much research has been directed toward finding a link between emotional distress and obesity. Original studies conducted by scientists in the 1950s found a connection between anxiety and eating. It was therefore widely assumed that fat people ate because they were anxious. More recent work has failed to confirm consistent relationships between size, appetite, and emotions. Most contemporary investigators agree that at least one-third of all obese people eat the same or less food than their thinner peers.

Some recent research has revived speculation that anxiety, depression, and stress predispose some people for obesity (Figure 3-6). Reports from professional counselors and research scientists have described how people gain weight when they are upset and lose it again under stable life conditions. Some therapists see the use of food as a compensation for life's upsets, replacing what seems to be missing in life, and soothing, calming, and covering up daily stresses. But we know, too, that there are people who do just the reverse: they lose their appetites when they are troubled, sometimes becoming dangerously thin.

We have observed that people under stress have a tendency to do the opposite of what is good for them! Thin people stop eating, fat people go on binges. This is entirely consistent with the research on body types that we have discussed briefly above and refer

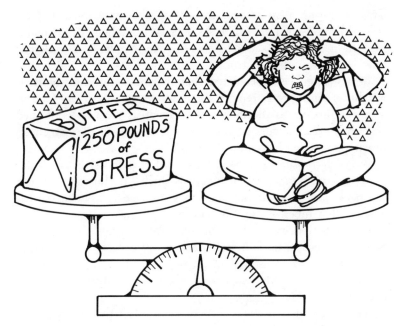

Figure 3-6. Stress sometimes equals weight gain.

to in more detail in Chapter 6. Soft, round, endomorphs seek comfort in food and human contact. Bony ectomorphs lose their appetites and retreat into isolation.

Other studies have suggested that obese people, especially obese women, use fat as a shield to hide behind. That is, the fat makes a statement to the world about what they can and cannot do. It may protect them from certain social and cultural obligations because few people expect a fat person to date or have an active sex life.

The fact that most obese people do, in fact, have normal sex lives, marry, and bear children, has barely dented the power of this widespread assumption. Many people still believe that being fat totally limits social opportunity. Heavy people are apt to be bombarded with unwelcome suggestions about how they could improve their fortunes.

"My mother and grandmother are pretty heavy, but my dad is very thin. He keeps telling me I wouldn't have to worry about dieting if I'd just run 35 miles a week like he does!"

Possible Physical Causes

Two promising areas of research on possible physical causes for obesity bear discussion. The first concerns how the body generates heat from food; the second concerns why metabolism is slowed down in certain obese persons.

It has long been speculated that mammals can control their weight by raising body temperature and burning off excess food in a process known as **thermogenesis.** Scientists recently confirmed that this indeed occurs and isolated the sources of thermogenesis in what are called brown fat deposits.

Brown fat, which is named for its color, is found in small deposits in rodents and other mammals, including humans, around the neck and chest. It has been most frequently associated with animals that hibernate and is known to play a role in survival at very low temperatures. Experimental data suggest that another function of brown fat is literally to burn off excess food so that it does not have to be stored in fat deposits. This can be accomplished by raising body temperature locally and radiating away unneeded energy.

This phenomenon could account for the fact that many people never alter their adult weight regardless of how much they eat. Heavy people appear to have less brown fat than average weight people, and what they do have seems to work inefficiently. Studies are under way exploring techniques that could increase thermogenesis and permit obese people to burn off their excess fat. We look forward to additional developments in this promising area of research.

The second fascinating new theory of obesity proposes that a deficiency of an enzyme with the strange name **ATPase** may predispose certain people to weight gain by lowering their resting energy expenditure by as much as 25 percent. Obese people typically have 20 to 25 percent less ATPase than do people of normal weight. The more obese the person is, the lower his or her concentration of ATPase is likely to be.

A consequence of these lower levels of ATPase is to alter caloric efficiency in favor of obese people, who burn fewer calories than normal weight people when they perform the same amount of activity.

The reason this happens seems to be related to an important metabolic process known as the **sodium pump,** which maintains different concentrations of sodium and potassium ions across certain cell walls throughout the body. It has been shown that obese people have lower pressure differentials across cell membranes than do normal weight subjects. This means that the sodium pump consumes less energy in obese people, who therefore survive on fewer calories.

These findings lend further credence to the claim of many overweight persons that they do **not** eat more than other, slimmer members of their families. This claim has found consistent support in public health studies conducted around the world over the past 20 years. Unfortunately, because these studies have contradicted our conventional wisdom, they often have been ignored. **Now, however, the evidence is too conclusive to ignore, and we can state that many obese people eat less than the nonobese, and that periodic dieting or fasting often has the long-term effect of making heavy people heavier.**

In the light of these developments, it seems we should revise our whole focus of attention. Since almost everyone in Western societies eats more than they need to survive, we should, instead of looking for why some people are fat, search for the mechanisms that keep most people thin. As scientists discover that heredity, fat cell deposits, hormone variations, thermogenesis, and other metabolic effects contribute to obesity, it becomes clearer that will power and morality are irrelevant in determining how much fat a person is destined to carry.

THE CONSEQUENCES OF OBESITY

"I am so tired of being judged first for my weight and second for my personality."

There are numerous consequences related to being overweight, most of them negative. In some cases, the more overweight one is, the more serious the consequences are. One generally inescapable handicap of obesity is prejudice. Surveys show that even fat people agree that being heavy is evidence of poor character. It is easy to see how that translates into self-critical attitudes.

Furthermore, some of the strongest social prejudices against fat people are held by health professionals who know how hard it is to change obesity. Surveys of physicians indicate that many of them view heavy people as lazy, self-indulgent, indifferent about their appearance, weak-willed, emotionally disturbed, or jolly slobs (slob defined as dirty, dumb, and lazy). Verbal harrassment of the obese is a frequently reported public occurrence. Even children are victimized.

Heavy children are less likely to be among the most popular in school, where athletics are often a social focus. Among young people, the norm of being pretty or muscular is very strong. Lack of ability to conform to these values may lead to ostracism and cause lasting emotional scars. Later, the obese person may find it particularly humiliating to be the one friend in a group of old friends who is not, for example, asked to be a member of a wedding party, who discovers that he or she is welcome only when the whole group gathers, and who is the last to find a partner when the gang grows up and pairs off.

Anne

At 5 feet 2 inches and 196 pounds, there was no question that Anne was a soft, round person! And a lively and attractive one, too. Anne was everyone's friend and nobody's lover. Men often sought her counsel and cried on her shoulder, but they never dated her. When she came to us for help, she was 30 and a virgin—a combination that depressed her and saddened us.

We offered support, warned her away from crash diets, and urged her to be patient. Since a trouble shared is a trouble halved, Anne felt better and regained some of her familiar spontaneity. She also joined a bowling league, where she was able to demonstrate convincingly that her shape did not impair her athletic ability. Six months later, when next we heard from her, we learned that she had improved her score both on and off the alley. She had a boyfriend she was delighted with, and she assured us repeatedly that he was well worth waiting for.

Anne's parents, who were also heavy, were fond of reminding her that they, too, had had a long search before they met. Judging by the snapshot she showed us of her boyfriend, if the relationship proves successful, Anne's own children will very likely face the same task of seeking acceptance as fat people.

Overweight seems to carry more serious social consequences for women. The following statement was made by Dr. Helen De Rosis at a seminar in Washington, D.C., entitled Overweight: Its Special Implications for Women: "A man, even if he weighs 250 to 300 pounds, does not incur the public adverse regard that a woman does. Men are supposed to be big. But women are not."

In recent years, heavy women have begun to recognize that the unfair discrimination they experience can be overcome. Fat consciousness raising groups have formed at many women's centers, and two glossy fashion magazines, *Big Beautiful Women* and *Radiance* (see Suggested Readings), have built up loyal and appreciative followings.

Nevertheless, it is still important to recognize that the physiological disadvantages of obesity, while they in no way warrant discriminatory attitudes, can be serious and, in some cases, life threatening.

For many years, excess weight has taken a comparatively greater physical toll on men than on women. But, because of the higher incidence of obesity in women, it is important to look further at the health complications unique to them. Women suffer not only from the general consequences; they also are reportedly subject to a variety of reproductive system difficulties: decreased fertility, increased likelihood of spontaneous abortions, prolonged and difficult childbirth, and general menstrual problems. Higher rates of uterine cancer also have been reported in obese women. And breast cancer is related to obesity in older women—certainly it makes detection more difficult.

As heavy people age, their weight may aggravate joint problems and create spinal problems, especially among women.

Obesity has been associated with some 26 medical conditions that may account for as much as 20 percent of the mortality rate. It has been related to increased incidence of hypertension, gallbladder disease, stroke, heart disease, and diabetes.

Association, however, is not the same as **cause.** Both age and baldness are associated with heart disease, but neither of them cause it; and turning back the clock or wearing a wig will not prevent it. We are not arguing that obesity is a desirable condition. It is not. But fat people should not be condemned or "treated" because of guilt by association.

Not all the consequences of obesity are negative. There is evidence that extra adiposity protects against common lung diseases—especially emphysema—and the overall cancer rate is lower in heavy people. Heart disease, which is frequently cited as a risk with obesity, may be more closely associated with hazardous weight loss treatments than with obesity itself. Epidemiological and animal studies strongly suggest that many cardiovascular problems, especially hypertension and congestive heart failure, occur with greater frequency among heavy people only because they strive repeatedly to lose weight.

SUMMARY

This chapter describes some of the varied popular views of overweight and obesity, and notes how difficult it is both to define and to measure obesity. The familiar Metropolitan Life tables of recommended weights are not representative of a healthy American average, nor of a long-lived minority; they list weights lower than most adults achieve.

Adiposity may consist of above average number of fat cells, above average sized fat cells, or both. Although there is no doubt about the social disadvantages of a fat or endomorphic body, the physical health hazards are less easy to assess. Obesity is to be avoided if possible without harmful dieting, and accepted if it is a genetic characteristic. Discrimination against fat people, though common, is unjustified and cruel, but there is little evidence that heavy people are less happy or successful than their lighter peers are.

CHAPTER REVIEW

◆ ──────── VOCABULARY ──────── ◆

adipose tissue fat tissues.

arousal state sense of intensity or anxiety.

ectomorphy tendency to be thin and bony.

endomorphy tendency to be soft and round.

mesomorphy tendency to be heavily muscled.

midrangers being near average on all three traits of endomorphy, mesomorphy, and ectomorphy.

obesity controversial term often taken to mean at least 20 percent above the weight recommended for one's height.

panacea cure for all ills.

postpartum depression a depression that follows childbirth in some mothers. Cases can be mild or severe enough to be labeled psychosis and require hospitalization.

serotonin neuro (brain) transmitter (message sender) that stimulates certain nerve cells to induce a feeling of calm. This may occur following the eating of carbohydrates, thus creating an analgesic or calming effect.

sodium pump body's method of maintaining different concentrations of essential ions (sodium and potassium) across cell membranes. The mechanism uses significant amounts of energy. Excess adiposity has been associated with reduced sodium pump function.

steatopygia large buttocks and heavy upper thigh distribution of fat deposits.

thermogenesis generation of heat, particularly in brown fat deposits, which provides necessary warmth, and may also be a way the body burns excess food and so avoids weight gain.

◆ ──────── FOR YOUR CONSIDERATION ──────── ◆

◆ People may be fat for different reasons. Describe a person you know who was born to be fat, and another who may be fat because of an unhealthy lifestyle. Be careful not to violate anyone's privacy. How do these people deal with their unfashionable appearance? Why do you think we attach so much importance to size and shape?

◆ What gender differences have you observed in the way society treats "overweight" men versus "overweight" women?

Who's at Risk
The Chance for Being Fat

This chapter will help you:

1. Understand the risk factors for obesity.
2. Describe the risk factors for anorexia and bulimia.
3. Demonstrate knowledge of rating charts for the above risk factors.

◆

*"I wanted someone to see
what I was doing and say,
'STOP!' But no one
noticed, so on I went."*

We now turn to a review of the populations that have a high risk for developing obesity and pathorexia.

Recent research has yielded some important concepts that must be considered if obesity and eating disorders are to be prevented. To begin with, we can better understand the problem by examining two separate groups: those with adult-onset obesity and those with juvenile-onset obesity.

The juvenile-onset obese are defined as people who have become at least 20 percent above the average weight during infancy or adolescence.

This percentage is 10 percent less than the value used in defining obesity in Chapter 3, and thus may include some heavy individuals who could not, by our definition, be considered obese. Yet 20 percent is used here because we are working with the definition of obesity that is most generally accepted in the medical community. This is not an easy statistic to discover, because children's heights and weights are even more variable than those of adults. Most of us, however, believe we know what we mean when we describe a child as fat.

There appear to be three main factors leading to juvenile obesity. The first contributing factor is **heredity.** The child of one obese parent has a 40-percent chance of becoming obese; the risk increases to 80 percent if both parents are obese (Figure 4-1).

Figure 4-1. Heredity and body type play a role in the risk for being fat.

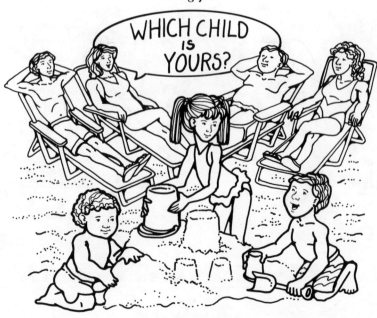

The second factor that appears to contribute substantially to juvenile-onset obesity is **early overnutrition.** Fat babies may be called cute, and mothers may get compliments about how "healthy" their babies look, but a rotund baby is far from a picture of good health. In actuality, the weight put on during infancy is likely to predispose an individual to a lifetime of being overweight.

The third contribution to early weight gain relates to **emotions.** When we pacify babies with bottles and young children with sweets, they soon learn to adopt this type of behavior on their own. If a baby cries or a child takes a fall and we respond by comforting the child with something sweet, it should not surprise us to find this same child coming home from an upsetting day at school and cleaning out the refrigerator. Stress and anxiety continue to rank among the most plausible contributors to weight gain in both juvenile- and adult-onset groups.

CAUSES OF OBESITY

We will examine the causes of obesity in two separate groups based on age of onset, because juvenile obesity influences an individual's physiology for the rest of his or her life.

Although obesity is a widely researched area, until the 1970s few investigators focused on age of onset as a critical issue for their studies. This is due, in part, to the relatively recent discovery of the relationship between juvenile-onset obesity and the production of fat cells. A critical time for the development of fat cells occurs between birth and age two. A second period begins in early adolescence. The number of fat cells produced during these periods is related to heredity, nutrition, and activity level.

Early-onset (juvenile) obesity is associated with an increase in cell numbers. In most cases, adult-onset obesity represents simply an enlargement of already existing cells. Once one has become an adult, new fat cells are developed only in response to massive overfeeding for a prolonged period of time. A juvenile-onset obese individual who loses weight continues to have more adipose cells than those who have never been overweight, and more than those who have become heavy for the first time as adults.

Decreases in the body fat of juvenile-onset obese individuals are accompanied by a reduction of cell size but no changes in cell number. Dr. Judith Rodin, an international authority on obesity, writes: "Thus, even in children, once a particular adipose cell number is achieved, it cannot be decreased by dietary restriction, and these (one-time fat) children usually become overweight adults."

The significance of the number of fat cells cannot be overemphasized. It appears that fat makes fat. The larger and more numerous one's adipose cells are, the greater becomes the ability of the body to produce and store more fat. This means that **people who are substantially overweight have a greater risk of further weight gain than do normal weight individuals.** The more cells one carries, the greater is one's physiological predisposition to fat. And remember that the number of cells cannot be diminished.

When examining the etiology (cause) of adult-onset obesity, the first suspect is always juvenile-onset obesity. Was this person actually an obese infant or child who is simply returning to an enlarged state as programmed by her or his fat deposits? If the individual is truly overweight for the first time, we then look for other causes.

One factor that appears to contribute significantly to obesity is conscious appetite restraint, or rather the removal of such restraint. Many people constantly, actively, and consciously resist food. Under certain circumstances, their motivation to resist is reduced—marriage, pregnancy, and depression are frequently cited examples—and control of eating is essentially lost. Thus, a woman who has been at normal weight all her life may become obese during pregnancy, not only because the pregnancy changes her metabolism, but also because the knowledge that her figure will soon become enlarged no matter what she eats gives her permission to abandon restraint in eating.

Stress, anxiety, and depression have repeatedly been assumed to have a direct relationship to adult-onset obesity. In our own research, however, we have found that the only emotional handicap linked fairly consistently to obesity is depression, and even that is by no means a universal connection.

There are also complex interrelationships between obesity and one's socioeconomic status, race, and ethnic origin. About one-third of all lower socioeconomic status adults have been identified as obese, compared with only one in twenty upper status women and less than one-fifth of upper status men. According to scientists who study populations, black women of low socioeconomic status are at the greatest risk of all. Roughly 50 percent of them have skinfold measurements above the 85th percentile for women in general.

We suspect that poverty, cultural values, and cultural changes all have an impact on weight. Poor immigrants (including poor blacks who move to northern cities) who are exposed to relatively inexpensive, high-calorie food may increase their intake. Obesity

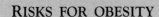

RISKS FOR OBESITY

High Risk of Obesity: *Juvenile-onset*

1. Being female
2. Parent(s)/Grandparents obese
3. Overfeeding in infancy
4. Excessive use of food to cope with stress or as a reward for achievement

High Risk of Obesity: *Adult-onset*

1. History of juvenile obesity
2. Being female
3. Parent(s)/Grandparents obese
4. Long-term depression or stress
5. Long-term history of restrained eating
6. Massive overeating for a sustained period of time
7. Low socioeconomic status
8. First or second generation American or subject of major cultural change

may thus be induced in those of them who are physically at risk. Cultural values in these populations may not include prejudice against being overweight or obese—indeed, a soft roundness in a woman and heaviness in a man may be viewed positively.

Also, cultural change may result in the loss of healthful, traditional dietary customs that are replaced by the seductive messages of advertisements for processed food. The impact of all these factors diminishes with assimilation and education.

The accompanying chart summarizes the risks for obesity and includes factors discussed both in this chapter and elsewhere in this book.

The accompanying brief questionnaire summarizes and weighs the severity of certain risk factors for obesity. The interpretation that follows provides a general sense of whether a tendency to become obese exists. Those who score over 16 points but who are not now obese should take all precautions necessary to prevent obesity from developing.

RATE YOUR RISK OF OBESITY

Give yourself:

1. 5 points for each obese parent or − 10 if neither was obese _____ pts.

2. 5 points if you are a moderate social drinker _____ pts.

3. 15 points if you were fat as an infant or adolescent, − 15 if you have never been heavy _____ pts.

4. 5 points if you frequently turn to food when upset _____ pts.

5. 5 points if you frequently feel depressed _____ pts.

6. 5 points if life has recently been unusually stressful _____ pts.

7. 5 points if your life revolves around restraining your appetite (constant dieting) _____ pts.

8. − 10 points if you exercise four or more times in a week _____ pts.

total points _____

Scoring and Interpretation

−35—0 points: It is highly unlikely that you will develop fat.
1—15 points: There is a minor chance that you will have a weight problem.
16—25 points: You have a modest tendency toward becoming overweight.
26—40 points: You are at considerable risk for becoming overweight.
41—50 points: You are in the high risk group.

Pathorexia—severely disordered appetite—is most frequently a disorder of childhood and adolescence that primarily affects females. The conforming, undemanding, and unassuming child is often the victim. Such children seem as though they cannot do enough to please their parents and are typically attractive and good students—too good for their own good.

Pathorexic children are good because they feel insecure. A common reason for developing the disorder is a conscious or unconscious effort to keep a disintegrating family together. Pathorexia creates a problem that parents can work on together, thus stalling the family discord that the child fears so much.

ANOREXIA, BULIMIA, BULIMAREXIA

"I couldn't leave the house for any reason without giving myself an enema first!"

Diane

Diane's anorexia began imperceptibly shortly after her parents started to talk about divorce. Never anything but thin, Diane had still not entered puberty at 14. Even she did not realize that she was skipping meals and spending hours staring into space.

Finally, when she had dropped to 56 pounds, a teacher brought her parents' attention to the problem. Her mother and father recognized that Diane was starving herself to death and hospitalized her.

Diane's depression, which had caused her loss of appetite, gave way to anorexia during the hospitalization. She was a difficult, disruptive patient at first, but began to eat after two months of family counseling. Her parents always came and left the counseling sessions together, and they increasingly supported each other's attitudes and opinions.

Only in retrospect did Diane and her family recognize that her crisis had been the beginning of the parent's reconciliation.

Sometimes children feel compelled to behave in an overly conformist fashion because they sense that one or both of their parents need them to be well-behaved to maintain the parents' shaky convictions about the right way to live.

When this happens, the child becomes a parental figure. This can easily create a stress overload in an already insecure youngster. The good child also frequently reports not knowing how to cope with the give-and-take of peer relationships. The child can only respond to others by playing strictly by the rules.

Many pathorexics are unable to express anger effectively, especially toward a parent or an authority figure. In most households, adolescence is associated with a difficult shift of authority from parents to maturing children. In disordered families, there may be little overt evidence of conflict, anger, or a desire for new experiences. Instead, the child's disordered appetite becomes a metaphor for other appetites: fear of and desire for sexual expression, fear of and desire for closeness in relationships with others (especially parents), or fear of and desire to simply let go of all emotions, be they joyful, angry, or just loud! Often the family has the outward appearance of being the epitome of middle class normality.

"My mother is such a great lady. I can't believe I'm telling you I hate her now. But when I think of all the ways she made my life so perfect, so soft, so cushie, I get furious. Now I can't handle anything by myself. I don't even know who I am!"

Sometimes, however, it is the complete absence of middle class norms that causes a child to become the family caretaker.

Gretchen

Gretchen's parents divorced when she was an infant. Her mother, a talented musician, helped make ends meet by singing in nightclubs and bars. Unfortunately, her career was handicapped by her tendency to get drunk. Gretchen's childhood was terrorized by the men her mother brought home, some of whom made sexual advances toward Gretchen.

Gretchen resolved that she would grow up to be everything her mother was not. She was a model child at home—cleaning, cooking, and maintaining her room spotlessly. She was an excellent student, and worked hard to become a good pianist. But she could not overcome her fear and disgust of men and of physical contact of any kind.

Gretchen became bulimic after she got a job at a doughnut shop. Her fellow workers were very social, held parties often, and dated among themselves. Gretchen could not bring herself to join in the fun. Instead, she took home boxes of day-old doughnuts and binged alone in her room. The more isolated she felt, the more she turned to food for comfort—starving herself for three or four days after each binge to avoid weight gain.

Examining the family life of pathorexics often reveals intelligent and capable mothers who gave up their career aspirations to be excellent parents. This struggle for excellence, they reasoned, could be measured by the proper development of their children. To experience success, such well-intentioned mothers become enmeshed in all aspects of their daughters' lives.

Fathers, on the other hand, are typically immersed in their own careers and remain emotionally distant. Nevertheless, even though he may express them only rarely, the father's values have a powerful impact on the family. For example, if a child overhears the father commenting on the mother's expanding waistline, the remark, though lightly intended, may register in the teenager's mind as an imperative to stay slim.

Two dynamics with negative consequences can thus be set in motion for the teenage child. First, the child must be thin to avoid Dad's disapproval. Then, in remaining thin, there is direct competition with the mother, a state that neither parent nor child is likely to miss.

Although Dad's comments may have been intended as helpful or were benign, they generate both fear and hostility in children, and they do nothing positive for Mother's ego! The children may feel more isolated and more in conflict about their roles as young adults and about their status within the family. Always chronic pleasers, the children are in a no-win situation.

"I know if I didn't get good grades, my folks wouldn't say anything, but they sure are happy with my straight A's. I hope I never disappoint them."

About-to-be pathorexic children feel that their activities are controlled, whereas their emotions are ignored. Their secret life with food is a metaphor of, an escape from, and a rebellion against the barrenness of their lives. They compensate by bingeing, purging, and starving until they are discovered or allow themselves to be caught. (Some bulimics "forget" to flush the vomitus in their parents' bathroom bowl.)

The discovery that their child is pathorexic may have a convulsive effect on the family, especially when the child must be hospitalized. We have likened it to a delayed action bomb that has been ticking away for months or years and finally explodes, exposing the family to a danger that has been present, but ignored, for a long time.

DANGER SIGNS: PATHOREXIA IN PROGRESS

1. Binge eating, no eating, or secretive eating
2. Withdrawal from friends and all social activities, or an obvious preference for friends who are themselves eating disordered
3. Obvious change in eating patterns
4. Constant preoccupation with food—cooking and shopping for others
5. Frequent, frenzied, and excessive exercise
6. Evidence of forced vomiting; frequent use of laxatives, diuretics, or enemas
7. Rapid change in weight, especially weight loss

Besides the need to be good and to function only by the rules, pathorexic children demand perfection from themselves. The obsession with thinness and the fear of fat are part of a determination to maintain a perfect record of control, proving to themselves that they can manage everything they feel responsible for. Through "constructive starvation," they sublimate both their fear of failure and their anger at a world that demands so much of them while giving them little in return.

The profile of a child at high risk for pathorexia includes the following:

1. Being female
2. Being undemanding, even from infancy
3. Consistently achieving excellent grades
4. Never talking back to parents
5. Showing limited emotional expression, especially of anger
6. Having parents obsessed with appearance/perfection
7. Living in a home where there is marital discord or alcohol abuse, or living with the fear of losing a parent through illness
8. Experiencing a severe setback in personal or interpersonal goals
9. Hanging out with a number of friends already known to be eating disordered
10. Becoming ritualistic and obsessive about food

RATE A CHILD'S RISK OF PATHOREXIA

Give the child:

1. 10 points if female, − 10 if male ___10___ pts.

2. 5 points if he or she has always been undemanding and cooperative ___5___ pts.

3. 5 points if he or she is generally a perfectionist, adding another 5 points if his or her appearance must always be perfect, and adding another 5 if his or her school grades must always be perfect. Subtract 5 if your child is willing to "let some things go," and subtract another 5 for less than perfect appearance or grades ___−10___ pts.

4. 5 points if he or she expresses little or no anger ___0___ pts.

5. 10 points if either you or your spouse has been ill, missing from home, or incapacitated for a prolonged period of time ___10___ pts.

6. 10 points if you and your spouse are currently having, or have recently experienced, marital problems ___0___ pts.

7. 10 points if he or she has recently experienced a traumatic event such as a move away from friends and school or if he or she has been abused or sexually harassed; give 20 points if both have occurred ___10___ pts.

8. 10 points if there is a history of obesity in the family; − 10 if there is no history of such ___−10___ pts.

9. 10 points if he or she often struggles to lose weight ___0___ pts.

10. 5 points each if either you or your spouse is preoccupied with food or physical appearance (this could total 20 if both parents are preoccupied with food and appearance.) ___0___ pts.

11. 5 points if he or she frequently speaks of hating his or her body ___5___ pts.

total points ___20___

Scoring and Interpretation

−35—0	points:	Pathorexia highly unlikely
1—25	points:	Little likelihood of pathorexia
26—56	points:	Moderate risk
57—87	points:	High risk
88—120	points:	Expect to see danger signs

SUMMARY

This chapter reviews several major risk factors for obesity, which include: female gender, genetics, overfeeding, high stress, a personal history of obesity, restrained eating, and low socioeconomic status. These risk factors are divided into juvenile-onset and adult-onset categories of weight gain.

The second section of this chapter examines risk factors for pathorexia, which include: female gender, passivity, obsession with appearance, perfectionistic goals, and maintenance of an eating disordered peer group. These risk factors and those for obesity are evaluated in terms of their cumulative influence on the onset of a problem.

CHAPTER REVIEW

◆ ──────── VOCABULARY ──────── ◆

adult-onset   occurring for the first time in those who have reached maturity.

diuretic   chemical that stimulates the production of urine. Also known as a water pill.

enema   a liquid forced into the lower bowel through the rectum to compel elimination.

etiology   cause.

juvenile-onset   occurring from infancy to young adulthood.

sublimate   expression of an "unacceptable" impulse in a positive or acceptable way.

◆ ──────── FOR YOUR CONSIDERATION ──────── ◆

◆ Review the health risks for obesity and eating disorders. Which do you think are the most significant factors? Can you list additional factors?

◆ In this chapter eating disorders and obesity are related to family problems. Why do you think children and teenagers use food to express their distress? Why are girls at greater risk than boys? Do adults in troubled families also abuse food? Are children or adults more likely to abuse food? List reasons for your answers.

AVOIDING TROUBLE
Prevention Is Better Than Cure

This chapter will help you:

1. Understand the difficulties and resistance of pathorexia to "cure."
2. Describe a rationale for preventive measures.
3. Implement preventive strategies.

◆

"If only I hadn't started bingeing and purging. I feel like an addict. Even when I'm eating normally and not vomiting, I feel like it's lurking right over my shoulder waiting to snare me again."

Both obesity and pathorexia are resistant to cure once they have a firm hold on an individual. They may be emotionally and physically hazardous diseases, and some of the known treatments carry substantial risks with only limited results. This chapter presents a case for the prevention of obesity and pathorexia and makes some suggestions on how to accomplish those goals.

Appetite disorders are a serious concern to literally millions of Americans. Severe obesity is linked to hypertension, diabetes, cardiovascular disease, increased risk of cancer, aggravation of degenerative joint diseases, and economic and social handicaps. There is overwhelming evidence that a person who once becomes obese will remain so. Those who do reduce fight a continuous battle with food and often return to the obese state.

WHY PREVENTION IS THE BEST ANSWER

> "Every time I sit down to a meal, something inside of me makes me feel like this is my last chance to be full, so I tell myself, 'Go eat all you can.'"

The act of dieting itself appears to be an emotionally difficult endeavor. Depression, irritability, anxiety, and hostility are reported much more frequently in dieters than in nondieters, regardless of whether they are obese or of normal weight.

Cure after cure has failed the obese person, with weight loss nearly always being followed by substantial weight increase. Even radical surgical interventions that shorten the intestine or reduce the size of the stomach cannot make good a lasting guarantee of slimness. In addition, the risk of complications—such as diarrhea, malnutrition, liver disease, bacterial overgrowth, kidney failure, arthritis, and choking—make such measures far from ideal.

The pathorexic faces at least equivalent risks (Figure 5-1). Death through self-imposed starvation is certainly the supreme loss, with the risk of heart disorders from potassium imbalance an ever present possibility. Further risks include all the physical symptoms related to malnutrition, including kidney disease, menstrual problems, metabolic changes, and mood swings. Additional complications that are a direct result of purging behaviors include stomach ruptures, the inability to defecate without external stimulation, sore throats, tooth decay, scarred hands from pressure exerted during forced vomiting, diseased and swollen salivary glands, and small bruises from burst blood vessels around the eyes.

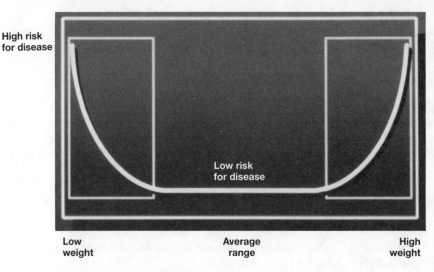

Figure 5-1. *Health risks increase at extreme underweight and extreme overweight.*

The depression, irritability, and anxiety found in obese populations while they diet becomes a way of life for pathorexics. Their distorted body image may keep them in a constant state of near panic. They live their lives for food. They plan their days around food—either how to get it or how to avoid it. It is a true full-time obsession.

Statistics on "cure" rates for pathorexia are not readily available. The National Association of Anorexia Nervosa and Associated Disorders (known as ANAD) estimates that only 50 percent of all recovered pathorexics will remain free of symptoms, 25 percent will live with reduced behavior problems, and 25 percent will not experience any meaningful remission following therapy. These figures agree with our own results and thus point to a severe and lasting problem that we would rather prevent than treat. It may be helpful to think of the recuperating pathorexic as we think of the nondrinking alcoholic—in a state of recovery but always vulnerable, unable to ignore the potential for a return to the substance abuse, either food or drink.

The prognosis for the obese to remain permanently at a normal weight is bleak. The hope for a totally normal life for the pathorexic is guarded. It is clear, then, that the best case for prevention lies in the failure of available restorative therapies—a topic we will examine in more detail in later chapters.

"I started by only vomiting up the junk foods and letting three meals a day digest. Then I thought, wouldn't it be great to lose weight faster? If I had only known before I began what a mess I was getting into . . . ."

The first step toward prevention is to identify the populations at greatest risk. Parents, educators, therapists, physicians, dietitians, and other professionals can then work together to short circuit the mechanisms that promote these pernicious disorders.

MOVING TOWARD PREVENTION

Although large gaps remain in our understanding of why obesity and pathorexia develop, we do know enough to design profiles of high risk groups. If these problems are a result of how we live and what we expect from ourselves and our children, controlling them may lie in altering our lifestyles and expectations before we are stricken.

At the same time, it is important not to ignore the low-risk population. While reliable figures are not available, psychologists suspect that increasing numbers of men are becoming trapped in pathorexic addiction. Middle age, normal weight men who are anxious to regain or maintain their youthful silhouettes are developing anorexic, bulimic, and bulimarexic symptoms as they fight the battle of the bulge.

There is much evidence that our society's values with respect to weight and shape have become more rigid and critical in the last two decades. Although various kinds of body shapes have been fashionable in the past and women have felt it vital to their well-being to conform to fashion, only recently have a great many Americans felt the crushing passion to live by the norms of haute couture.

Barbara "Babe" Paley, the socialite wife of the former president of the Columbia Broadcasting System, coined the phrase, "You can never be too rich or too thin." The slogan caught on, despite the well-publicized fate of the billionaire Howard Hughes, who died alone in a state of extreme emaciation.

A century ago, Mrs. Paley's influence would not have extended beyond the tiny minority of the leisured rich. Today, her slogan is the watchword of tens of millions of Americans. The media constantly reinforce it by insisting that virtually everyone in movies and on TV be ectomorphic, regardless of the content of the film or program, creating the impression that only thin people are normal and only thin people can be successful or interesting.

On the other hand, we live in an economy that has a huge stake in selling us things we don't really need, including food. The food industry's profits depend on marketing processed food so tastily and attractively packaged and advertized that we will add it to our diet.

The conflict between the pressure to eat and the pressure to be thin has been heightened in recent years by the shift in our perception of the ideal American woman from images of apple pie and motherhood to a "supermom" capable of handling both career and family responsibilities. This expansion of women's roles has clearly aided women by enlarging their opportunities, but it has also increased the stresses on them.

Women are expected to be disciplined, authoritative, and in some cases "masculine" when they are at work, but they are expected to remain feminine and yielding in sexual and social settings.

The thin woman is thought to be best equipped for this dual role. With the minimally developed curves of her straight body, she wears the executive three-piece suit most successfully. For social occasions, she can switch to frilly fashions that exemplify the decorative side of her identity. Missing here is the acceptance of the full, soft, adult female form that many women are genetically ordained to inherit.

For preventive measures to be effective, powerful social and economic forces will have to change, with a primary focus on children's nutritional education. Teachers in all the grades and educators of future teachers and health professionals must pay attention to the principles of sound nutrition and healthy exercise. Parents, teachers, and therapists must avoid food-centered reward systems for dealing with stress or disappointment. ("If you'll stop crying, you can have a sucker.") They must learn, too, not to use sweets or junk food as rewards for good behavior either (Figure 5-2).

Health maintenance issues must be marketed for children in a way that competes successfully with the glamorous images that are projected for junk food and exercise-free entertainment. Health professionals need to develop models that teach good nutrition in new ways, ways that increase compliance among consumers. Families aware of the risks of overnutrition, underexercise, and overachievement are well set to cope with the legacy of 20th century affluence.

PREVENTIVE STRATEGIES

Unfortunately, a number of the risk factors for appetite disorders and obesity cannot reasonably be altered. With regard to obesity, if one is or has a female child with a familial history of being overweight, certain precautions are recommended. Special care

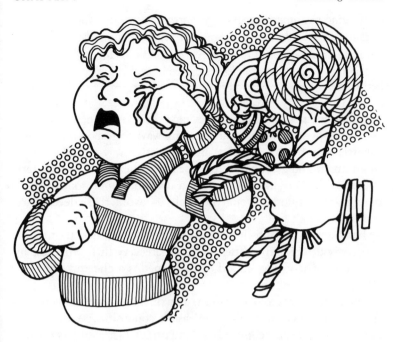

Figure 5-2. *Comforting a child with food creates a serious risk for obesity.*

should be taken to be sure that infants are neither overfed or underfed. Overfeeding produces additional fat cells that the individual will never be able to get rid of and that will always be ready to store unneeded surplus fat. Underfeeding may produce a pathorexic response that will result in the starving child being unable to control his or her appetite and being constantly obsessed with food.

Maria

Maria, an obese 30-year-old patient, had begun her constant search for snacks and sweets at about age three. But she had no idea why. She learned why during a Thanksgiving dinner with her family, when the conversation turned to reminiscing about early childhood. Maria's mother told how she had put Maria to bed with a glass bottle every night until she was two and a half. One night the bottle was broken in a mishap that soaked the mattress and left jagged glass in the bedding. The nightly bottle in bed ceased abruptly.

Hearing that anecdote was a watershed in Maria's life. From
that time on, she had a reason to resist overeating that
crystallized her desire to be grown up and in charge of her life.
She lost weight and stabilized at a comfortable weight.

When infants cry or children scrape their knees, parental attention and physical affection are healthy ways to respond. Although
a bottle may be the quickest, most effective way to induce quiet
in an infant and a cookie restores peace in the house, as long-term
strategies they are likely to induce a dependence on food. Parents
of high-risk children would do well to avoid these feeding responses.

Finding positive substitutes for food is the healthiest training we
can give our children. When children are very little, the best intervention when they are sad or frightened is a cheerful smile and
a hug.

As children get older, parents can involve them in activities
that distract them from the unpleasant conditions. Avoiding the
use of food for such coping is an important first step toward preventing overweight in children; using physical activity as a preferred outlet is a further step toward good health. Such activities
keep children away from food and have the advantage of burning
up calories.

Obese parents face a double bind. Not only are their children
in a high-risk group, but they themselves may wish to change any
established behavior patterns that may have contributed to their
own obesity and so avoid negative modeling for their children. We
acknowledge with respect the courage and determination it takes
for a heavy mother to involve her children in health promoting
athletic activities and dietary habits when she was never encouraged to do so herself.

Those who are at high risk for adult-onset obesity should take
precautions toward maintaining a state of good health (Figure
5-3). A woman with either family or a personal history of obesity
should not assume that during pregnancy she can "eat for two"
without a risk of unwanted weight gain. She needs to pay special
attention to maintaining a healthy pregnancy weight, both for the
fetus and for herself.

Too little weight gain robs both the mother and the fetus of
necessary nutrition and may actually cause deformities in the fetus
and lower the potential intelligence of the child. With too much
weight gain, the mother may have a difficult pregnancy or a difficult delivery, and may have a problem with weight control in the
future.

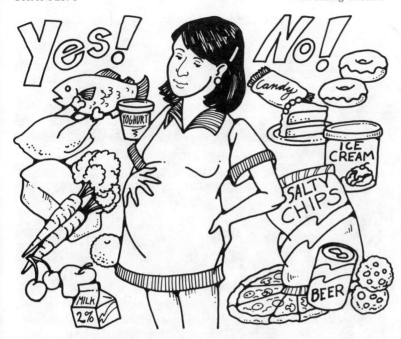

Figure 5-3. *Practicing prevention, especially during high-risk times, reduces the risk of obesity.*

Toxemia is also a frequent problem for women who gain too much weight. Pregnant women should keep in mind that pregnancy is a time when fat cells can emerge and become permanent additional tissue.

Those people who maintain their weight through continuous restraint or a lifetime pattern of avoiding certain foods know that an extended break from that restraint is likely to lead to obesity.

Restrained eaters seem to become trapped in a dilemma that permits no pleasant alternatives. They must always hold back or become fat. It may be that restrained eaters are actually fighting their natural or hereditary physiques. We discuss the importance of accepting hereditary characteristics as a preventive measure for pathorexia as well as for obesity throughout this book. For perpetual dieters, we offer the suggestion that **relaxed restraint,** which minimizes total prohibitions but always monitors intake of appetite provoking treats, may allow them to maintain better long-term control (Figure 5-4, p. 72).

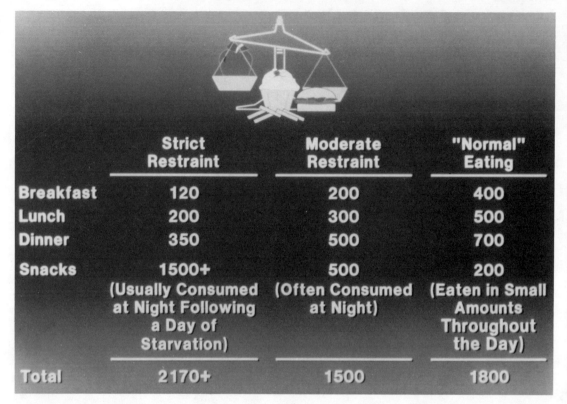

	Strict Restraint	Moderate Restraint	"Normal" Eating
Breakfast	120	200	400
Lunch	200	300	500
Dinner	350	500	700
Snacks	1500+ (Usually Consumed at Night Following a Day of Starvation)	500 (Often Consumed at Night)	200 (Eaten in Small Amounts Throughout the Day)
Total	2170+	1500	1800

Figure 5-4. *Strict restraint leads to increased calories.*

When they are depressed or must face stressful circumstances, women in high-risk groups appear likely to gain unwanted weight. Awareness of these dangerous times helps make it easier to fend off overeating. For high-risk people who are experiencing a great deal of stress, it may be wise to seal the refrigerator or take other precautions that will remind them that right now food is hazardous to their health!

Those who face this problem must prepare to cope with stress in ways that do not involve eating. Possibilities include seeking counseling, taking assertiveness training, running, swimming, even shopping for clothes. These are established techniques that work well, both alone and in combinations.

The pathorexic child is harder to identify in terms of predicting risk. As we mentioned earlier, pathorexia is most often a problem for girls. Parents who have a "perfect" daughter who never confronts them or disappoints them often find it difficult to question her about her health or their role as parents. Her record of exemplary behavior protects her like a shield from any implication that problems may exist. This tendency toward goodness, however, may be the first clue to the presence of turmoil beneath the surface.

An adolescent anorexic who was trying to survive on a regimen of lettuce and catsup told us, "When I was in second grade, we had to sit with our hands together. I used to imagine myself being perfectly still, not moving a muscle, and getting hundreds on all of my tests. I still think about that when I'm tempted to skip on my diet."

Permitting a child to be less than perfect is healthy. It is fine to have goals and dreams for children, but it is not fine to push those ideals on a child who does not fight back. It is not a good idea to decide what a child should become and then set out to control the child's life so that narrow dream can come true.

Mary

Mrs. Reed's first three children had always seemed destined for success. Sure enough, two became doctors, like their father and uncle, and the third became an architect. Mary, the fourth and youngest child, never had the energy or drive her brothers and sister had. Mrs. Reed decided that Mary would never leave home or marry. Mary would always be with her.

She subtly discouraged Mary's obvious talent for math and science while constantly reinforcing her artistic ability and rewarding her domestic skills.

When we met Mary at age 25, she had lived two lives for eight years. Outwardly demure, restrained, and conforming, she sincerely believed that her mother needed her to help look after her now sickly father. She had never learned to drive and was a prisoner in her own home.

Mary's second life was lived in her bedroom. There, she submerged her consciousness in a never changing world of

PREVENTING PATHOREXIA IN CHILDREN

"I guess I was just stupid. One time I forgot to flush the toilet and my mother saw the, you know, vomit. After that, she asked me a whole lot of questions, and finally I had to tell her the truth."

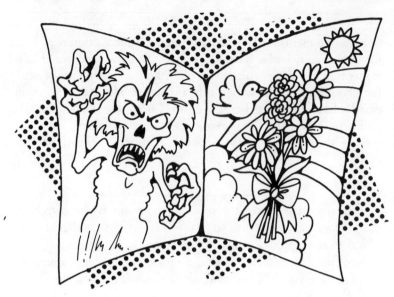

Figure 5-5. *The two extreme sides of Mary.*

science fiction novels and bulimarexic behavior. She used garbage bags to sneak vast quantities of food into her room and reused them to sneak the vomitus out, dumping them in the trash barrels of an apartment building next door. When she was not eating or reading, Mary made delicate, handcrafted greeting cards, which she gave away or sold, and grotesque illustrations of maimed monsters, which she kept for a while and then destroyed (Figure 5-5).

We suspect that Mary's mother knew more about her daughter than she ever admitted. But both of them had become victims of the mother's desire to have Mary stay home. Mary had failed to develop the social skills necessary to survive in the outside world, and her mother was so dependent on Mary's presence that she sabotaged every move her other children made to help their sister grow up.

There are three parental curses that are often innocently inflicted on children: the admonition, "Just do your best;" the wish, "All we want is for you to be happy;" and the slogan, "If a thing's worth doing, it's worth doing well."

Each of these familiar bits of homespun wisdom can easily be interpreted by a susceptible young person as minimal expectations for daily life rather than goals. When this happens, children can come to believe that they must feel happy, work themselves to exhaustion, and do everything perfectly the first time. This combination induces severe stress and an almost certain sense of personal failure. Teaching a child to expect life to be a mixture of successes and disappointments is excellent preventive medicine for a gamut of disorders, not the least of which is pathorexia.

One or both parents of pathorexics are often preoccupied with physical appearances. Their children frequently feel they must strive continually to look attractive. All too often, they develop ideals based on photographs in fashion magazines that are totally unattainable outside of a studio. As a consequence, they begin to form erroneous ideas about their looks, often thinking of themselves as fat or deformed if they cannot fit into ultrasmall clothing.

Parental remarks—positive or negative—about a preteenager's appearance may not be in the child's best emotional interest. Simply telling a perfectionistic girl that she should "knock off a few pounds" can set up a pathorexic response. As Susan Wooley, an expert with an international reputation in this field, said on the Donahue show, "This is the first generation of Americans to be raised by Weight Watchers mothers."

"When I'm on a diet, I think about food all the time. I wake up thinking about breakfast. When that is done, I think about lunch for three straight hours, and on and on. I wish I could think about sex once in a while, like other people my age."

THE NUTS AND BOLTS OF NUTRITION

We close this chapter on prevention with some observations about responsible nutrition from infancy through adulthood. These observations are not intended to be comprehensive, but they are a guide to a way of thinking about food and eating that will help forestall problems in the future.

Mother's First Question— Breast or Bottle?

Many studies show that breast feeding is both safer and healthier for the baby than bottle feeding. For example, one study found that most bottle-fed babies were significantly overweight at six weeks. Further studies show good correlation between weight gain at six weeks and obesity at school age. These studies and others show the importance of breast feeding. However, if a baby must be bottle fed, here are some suggestions for healthier bottle feeding:

- Calculate the formula exactly.
- Weigh the baby.
- Avoid the temptation to add "just a little bit extra formula."

Measure the formula carefully. The quantity of powder in one scoop may vary depending on the method used to scoop the powder out of the can. The powder must not be compacted into the scoop. It should be poured loosely into the scoop until the scoop is full. Then, a knife edge should be used to level off the scoop. The common practice of bunching the powder on one side of the can and pressing against the scoop results in compacting of the powder. Using this technique could result in twice as much powder being used in the formula as specified. Excess formula also results from simply shaking powder off the scoop, leaving it slightly heaped rather than level.

These lax measuring techniques may not appear important, but they can be. If a bottle of formula contains twice as much powder as needed, it has twice the calories, and the baby is thus more likely to become obese.

Not to be precise about this seemingly trivial problem would be equivalent to an adult eating up to twice as much on a daily basis. However, the adult, as discussed previously, is not as likely to increase the number of fat cells as a baby. Babies are in the right growth phase to increase the number of fat cells, and thus be set up for a lifetime of obesity.

The exact amount of formula should be given to a baby, no more. Parents tend to feel that the baby needs a bottle whenever it cries. However, the baby may have colic, be uncomfortable, be hot or cold, or have gas, or may simply want to be loved.

When all else fails to quiet a crying baby, rather than giving a bottle of formula, try sugar water. Sugar enhances the taste of water and the baby will take this from the bottle. Sugar water contains fewer calories than formula. Plain water can be used, but it is seldom successful as babies generally do not like it. Make the solution with no more sugar than is needed to satisfy the baby to avoid getting the child hooked on sugar at an early age. Another alternative for calming a crying infant is to use a pacifier.

Much anxiety can be associated with breast feeding. A mother who is having the slightest trouble with breast feeding or feels the least bit insecure must obtain advice and support. It is not enough to say that everything will work out and not to worry.

The La Leche League is a nationwide self-help group which promotes breast feeding and is a valuable source of help and support. An obstetrician can provide the name of a local contact.

A common basic insecurity is that the baby is not getting enough milk and therefore the baby will not grow up to be healthy. However, this problem can be overcome by weighing the baby. Otherwise, simply await the results of the baby's four-week physical. If the baby's weight is within normal ranges, breast feeding should continue.

Another potential problem is that many parents believe that the sooner babies start eating solids the better. It is seen by the parents as a sign of progress, growing up, and maturity, and, therefore, reflects positively on the parents. However, this is false. It is not necessary to have a six-seek-old baby taking solids, nor it is desirable. Some parents may regard it as a status symbol that their two-month-old baby is eating all sorts of baby foods, but the results of this early introduction of solids may lead to obesity later in life, which is not a status symbol.

Babies should not be pushed to take solids, but they can be started on pureed vegetables, fruits, or cereals at about 6 months. If prepared at home, sugar, sweetening agents, and salt (common in regular canned foods and some commercial baby foods) can be avoided.

Feeding School Age Children

Many parents believe that excessive feeding of school age children has some special benefit. They feel that they are giving their children everything they can possibly give them. Some mothers feel that a rich diet may prevent colds or hold other inaccurate folklore beliefs. And some simply substitute food for real affection. Many folklore beliefs persist and are not easily eradicated. You may very well laugh at them, but when you are a part of that folklore, it may be difficult for you, as a parent, to know how to feed your children.

Folklore aside, there are many reasons why children eat fattening food. It may simply be a habit. For instance, one child may take a second helping and the other child may follow because of sibling rivalry. A child may eat in order to imitate an adult. A child may be given food in order to quiet a cry. Food may also sooth the uncomfortable or the bored. Food is frequently used as a reward or to make sure a child has a good night's sleep. A child may be fed because the parents like the look of a fat baby. Even if parents are not fond of the idea, grandparents may apply subtle pressure to make sure the child obtains extra food.

The mother of one of the authors told us that cream was very good for you because it was used in the treatment of tuberculosis.

What we suggest is that children should be well fed but without learning bad habits and consuming food high in calories. We recommend three meals a day and encourage eating at the table with the family if possible. A child should have enough to eat at mealtime and that should be sufficient. It is not really a loving thing to ply a child with candies, chocolates, cakes, cookies, ice cream, fruit juices, and soda between meals. An occasional treat is appropriate but to make this part of a daily routine is teaching the child bad habits.

Let us look at the new breed of so-called health foods briefly. Many of these are extremely high in sugar, e.g., granola bars. Just because a food is advertised as healthful does not mean that it is. Breakfast cereals may contain up to 60% sugar; fruit juices and drinks may be very high in calories. When thirsty, drink double-diluted fruit juice, non-caffeinated herbal teas with a smidgen of sugar, or a glass of water.

As another example, honey may appear to be more healthful than sugar, but it provides virtually the same number of calories as pure sugar and supplies very little else. The claim, therefore, that a food is healthy or a "healthfood" should be viewed with some caution.

The Issue of Caloric Density

Many foods are high in caloric density. These foods are called "junk foods" or "empty calorie foods." They include candy, chocolates, cakes, cookies, doughnuts, pastries, potato chips, corn chips, pretzels, crackers, soda, ice cream, honey, sugar, syrup, jams, and jellies. It is all very well to simply prohibit these foods, but what do we use in their place?

The most effective approach is to use a substitute, and to use it from a very early age, rather than prohibit a fattening food. For example, dry popped corn without the oil is an acceptable snack. Fresh fruit is not high in calories; unsweetened applesauce, rice cakes, plain yogurt, herbal iced tea, all of these can be used for snacks and treats.

Go to your kitchen and take inventory of all the snack foods in the cabinets and refrigerator. You may be surprised to find out how much "junk food" you have lying about.

For most persons in the United States, overfeeding, not malnutrition, is the primary food-related problem. Overfeeding can result from misconceptions and misinformation about food. For example, children are taught that eggs, butter, milk, and cheese are good for them and are needed to make their bodies grow. However, most of these dairy foods cause hardening of the arteries and raise cholesterol levels. From a health point of view, it is more desirable to use only skim milk and skim milk-based cheeses and yogurt.

We need to get away from the idea of telling children how everything makes their bodies grow healthy. Instead we should concentrate on showing children reasonable alternatives to junk food.

One good way to stimulate interest in different foods in children is to let them participate in food preparation. Discuss nutrition while preparing the meal. Have the child mix up some bananas and plain yogurt for the family dessert. This positive way of teaching is fun and healthy and sets a good example.

Many children show an interest in growing their own vegetables. Even if you have no land, you may be able to grow tomatoes, peppers, and chives indoors. Growing vegetables indoors or outside is another "hands on" way to help children develop an interest in the right foods and the right choices early on in life.

We have included on the following pages some questionnaires to help you, members of your family, and your friends evaluate how well you understand and implement some of the important aspects of nutrition we have just discussed.

Children in the Kitchen

SUMMARY

We have repeatedly observed that some diets actually cause eating disorders; we discuss this point in more detail in the next chapter. Diets that produce starvation increase the body's craving for food and cause people to lose their ability to detect appetite. Fashion magazines and dieting literature continuously market thinness to teenagers. Parents who want ideal children also give them the message, both verbally and nonverbally, that they are expected to be thin. If thin is in and stout is out, what do you do with a naturally rounded body? Why, starve it, of course!

Naturally plump children who have inherited their shapes may go to great lengths to distort their own bodies in order to comply with society's current norms. Self-starvation and purging behaviors that begin as dieting techniques set up a lifetime of obesity problems or pathorexia.

The message here is to accept ourselves as less than perfect and to be realistic about our own and our children's physical appearance, not attempting to change what nature has given us. Prevention rests on giving permission to find and experience healthy outlets for all appetites: for food, for love, for independence, for security, for expression, for solitude, and for caring and being cared for.

This view does not contradict what we stated concerning the prevention of the onset of obesity by taking appropriate precautions for high-risk groups. Simply stated, one should strive less for the stick-thin figure of a fashion model and substitute instead a healthful lifestyle. This means good nutrition, adequate exercise, and plenty of reinforcement of the notion that one's well-being comes from the pursuit of happiness and not from being a doll-like person, appreciated only for one's appearance.

INFANT CARE/PREVENTION STRATEGY QUESTIONNAIRE

Rate your strategy in infant care/prevention

1. Did you breast feed for 4 or more months?   Yes = −5   No = 0

2. If you breast fed for 4 or more months, did you wait at least until the 4th month to add food supplements (other than iron and fluoride)?   Yes = −3   No = +1

3. If you bottle fed, did you carefully calculate the number of ounces of formula needed each day?   Yes = 0   No = +1

4. Did you often put in an extra bit of formula "just in case"?   Yes = +2   No = 0

5. Did you often feed your baby jello-water?   Yes = +3   No = 0

6. Did you regularly force your baby to overeat at bedtime in order to get a full night's sleep?   Yes = +4   No = 0

7. Was your baby ever below the 30th percentile for weight?   Yes = +4   No = 0

8. Was your baby ever above the 90th percentile for weight?   Yes = +5   No = 0

9. Were you certain that the baby foods you used were controlled for fats, sugars, and salt?   Yes = −3   No = + 3

10. Were you proud that your baby was plump?   Yes = +5   No = 0

total points _____

Scoring and Interpretation

−11—0	You've given your baby the best possible chance of avoiding weight problems.
1—10	Very minimal risk may exist.
11—20	Use caution in the future.
21—28	Your baby is at high risk for developing weight problems.

CHILDHOOD CARE/PREVENTION QUESTIONNAIRE

Rate your strategy for early childhood care/prevention

1. Do you coerce children into cleaning their plates?   Yes = +3   No = 0

2. Do you insist that children take a second helping?   Yes = +3   No = 0

3. Do either Mom or Dad frequently overeat in front of the children?   Yes = +3 No = 0

4. Does the whole family regularly engage in an active sport or exercise?   Yes = −5 No = +2

5. Check all of the following conditions under which you offer your child food.
   a. to console when upset   +2
   b. to quiet when misbehaved   +2
   c. to relieve when bored   +2
   d. to reward when good   +2
   e. to compensate when you are busy   +2

6. Does your child spend more than two hours per day in front of the television?   Yes = +2   No = 0

7. Do you encourage your child to develop and maintain friendships?   Yes = −2   No = +2

total points _____

Scoring and Interpretation

−7—0	Your child has an excellent chance of avoiding weight problems.
1—9	Minimal risk may exist.
10—19	Take care to help avoid developing problems.
20—25	Your child is at high risk for weight problems.

ADULT-PREVENTIVE CARE QUESTIONNAIRE

Adults—Rate your own preventive care

1. Do you exercise regularly?   Yes = −3   No = 0

2. Do you snack on junk foods between meals?   Yes = +3   No = 0

3. Do you eat while watching television?   Yes = +1   No = 0

4. Do you have junk foods in your home?   Yes = +2   No = 0

5. Do you eat three meals a day?   Yes = 0   No = +1

6. Do you drink more than two alcoholic drinks a day?   Yes = +2   No = 0

7. Is your mother, father, brother, or sister more than 30% overweight?   Yes = +6
   No = 0

8. Do you drink more than two glasses of nondiet soda or fruit juice daily?   Yes = +1
   No = 0

9. Do you eat after seeing something delicious on television or in a magazine?
   Yes = +2   No = 0

10. Do you eat extra fiber? (Bran)   Yes = −1   No = 0

11. Have you ever been overweight?   Yes = +5   No = −2

12. Do you experience long periods of depression?   Yes = +5   No = −2

13. Do you find life highly stressful?   Yes = +5   No = 0

14. Do you regard intimacy as the most meaningful part of life?   Yes = −5
    No = +2

15. Do you regard food as the most meaningful part of your life?   Yes = +6   No = 0

total points _____

Scoring and Interpretation

−13—0	Congratulations, you are healthy.
1—15	You have a slight risk of developing problems with food.
16—30	Extreme caution is in order.
31—41	We suspect you already have problems with food.

CHAPTER REVIEW

◆ ——————————— VOCABULARY ——————————— ◆

cardiovascular disease illness of the heart or the veins and arteries.

degenerative joint disease deterioration at the juncture between two bones (knee for example).

haute couture high society fashions.

hypertension higher than normal blood pressure.

induce cause, set up.

pernicious harmful, perhaps fatal.

◆ ——————— FOR YOUR CONSIDERATION ——————— ◆

◆ On page 68 of this chapter a paragraph begins, "For preventive measures to be effective [in reducing the incidence of eating disorders], powerful social and economic forces will have to change. . . . " Identify policies, practices, and traditions in your school (e.g., only whole milk is currently available at lunch) which could undermine sound nutrition, healthy exercise, and positive self-acceptance for students and faculty. Discuss ways these "forces" could be changed for the better.

◆ What resources, energy, and skills would it take to form a support group for people trying to feel good about themselves just as they are? Can you think of how such a group would be received in your school? What specific purpose might it fill? What might it be called? Who do you think should and would join?

THE PHYSICAL CAUSES OF EATING DISORDERS

This chapter will help you:

1. Understand the physical factors affecting appetite and adiposity.
2. Know the importance of heredity in determining weight and shape.
3. Know that the digestive system and the brain affect appetite and eating behaviors, and that these systems often misinterpret voluntary dieting as enforced starvation.
4. Understand how the body's corrective mechanisms often reinforce eating disorders.

◆

"I'd rather throw up three times a day than end up looking like my parents!"

The next two chapters provide an explanation of the physical and psychological reasons why people develop appetite disorders. We begin with the physical changes that occur and that cause a choice of behavior to develop into an addictive disease.

In the process of gathering a body of knowledge on eating and appetite disorders, we have concluded that there are six major factors that contribute to human appetite. They interact with each other in ways that are complex and unique to each individual. The factors are: **heredity, fat deposits, metabolism, brain functions, learned behavior,** and **the environment.** When these forces are out of balance, appetite disorders can develop.

Medical and physical trauma are other factors that should be mentioned, although they are outside the scope of this book. There are glandular and hormonal disorders and certain brain dysfunctions that affect both appetite and metabolism. Many medications have an impact on appetite for people who are being treated for diseases unrelated to eating.

Some physical handicaps limit activity so much that obesity is almost inevitable.

Certain emotional disorders can also have a marked effect on appetite, even though they are only loosely associated with eating. The most important one is depression, a disorder characterized by feelings of helplessness, hopelessness, and sadness. Depression causes major appetite swings and as much as a five percent weight change a month. Typically, heavy people with depression gain weight, and light people lose, but there are many exceptions. Some people gain as they become depressed and then lose weight as the disorder deepens.

There is evidence that severe bulimia is a form of depression, and a few medical researchers have staked their reputation on this claim. We do know that medications helpful to depressed patients sometimes relieve bulimic symptoms, but there is much controversy and discussion among therapists about why this is so.

Other severe psychiatric disorders may also reveal themselves through pathorexic symptoms. When this is the case, bizarre eating behaviors are never the only signs of disorder. Other significant symptoms will also be evident.

Disabling psychiatric disorders require intensive therapy, most often beginning with hospitalization, during which careful diagnosis can be made. Treatment then addresses the underlying emotional disorder, not the external symptoms. The following case study is an example of a patient whose eating disorder was accompanied by a serious personality disorder.

FACTORS THAT CONTRIBUTE TO HUMAN APPETITE

Marla

At 20 years of age, Marla had been actively bulimic for six years. She had already made two suicide attempts.

Her self-destructive impulses caused her to sabotage any friendships that threatened her isolation. Her acts of violence against herself included cutting her feet with broken glass and intentionally burning her lips, fingers, and arms with cigarettes. She selected certain sores and kept them open for months at a time by picking off scabs as they formed.

Marla vomited into a plastic bag in her bedroom wastebasket at least three times a day. During the purging, she turned up her radio to mask the sounds. Following the purging, she would sneak the bag into the bathroom at the far end of the hall, empty it, and steathily return it to her bedroom. Sometimes other members of her large family kept the bathroom in constant use, forcing Marla to either hide the vomitus in her room or fling it from her second story window to escape detection.

It was after her second suicide attempt that Marla was brought to our attention. Her parents were totally unaware of Marla's many forms of self-abuse and only sought therapy for their daughter at the insistence of her doctor.

We worked with Marla for over two years. Progress was very slow and not very steady, but she did improve. She was hospitalized twice when crises overcame her.

Her family moved and Marla was referred to another therapist, who continued to work with her for three years. Finally, she was able to live without regular therapy. She remains on medication and attends a self-help group at least once a week.

Marla's recovery required the joint efforts of psychologists, psychiatrists, and hospital personnel. Working alone, none of her therapists could have helped her.

If you suspect that other medical or psychiatric problems are contributing to an appetite disorder, seek competent professional help. The STEM program described in Chapter 10 may help with moderate disorders, but it is not appropriate for severe ones.

Before we explain the underlying causes of appetite disorders, it may be helpful to review the nature of healthy appetite control. So far as we know, most people adjust their eating patterns to meet their needs with relatively little effort. Physical and psychological forces operate smoothly and effectively in a cooperative fashion.

There is some evidence that without nutritional education, children will consume too much sugar and fatty foods, but cultural norms help limit unhealthy excess for most people.

Even though food intake does not precisely match energy expenditure, a balance is maintained so that physical appearance or size in clothes does not alter appreciably. In addition, the balance occurs at a size and weight that allow optimal physical health to be achieved.

Like everyone else, healthy eaters experience the temptation to overindulge and overeat from time to time. But, for reasons that are not at all well understood, it takes little effort on their part to regain a healthy equilibrium. It is most probable that healthy people routinely eat more than is nutritionally necessary. Their metabolisms adjust to the excess to prevent unneeded weight gain. This ability to compensate is lost by people who force upon themselves a regimen of semi-starvation in order to alter their shape. The failure of these normal regulating mechanisms is the principal cause of pathorexia.

THE HEALTHY APPETITE

Part of the biological inheritance we receive from our parents is a set of genes that will decide for us the basic size and shape of our bones, muscles, and fat deposits. The circumstances in which we grow up can modify these proportions, but there are limits to the changes. To some degree, we all resemble our parents. Characteristic facial features and body builds typically identify family members in several generations. Similarly, the tendency to be heavy runs in families. It has been shown that there is an 80-percent chance that the children of obese parents will also become obese, **even if they are adopted at birth and raised by thin foster parents.**

THE ANATOMY OF APPETITE

Heredity

We *vividly recall a client who told us about his Jewish grandmother, who had been hidden in a cellar in France during World War II. Even though she survived on minimal rations for almost three years, she was still quite rounded when she emerged. This proved to be something of an embarrassment for her at the time, just as the same genetic tendency to obesity embarrassed her grandson, albeit under totally different and far less pressured circumstances.*

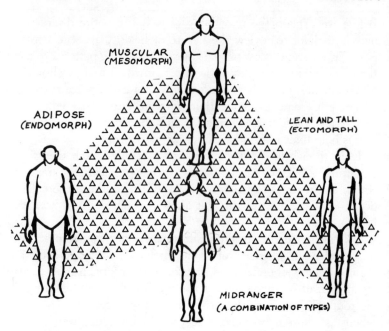

Figure 6-1. *The range of body types. All human bodies show varying degrees of adiposity, muscularity, and slenderness, and any body can be located within the triangle of body types.*

In this century, an American psychologist, William Sheldon, compiled the most comprehensive and scientific information on body types to date.

Based on an analysis of thousands of specially posed photographs, he derived a three-part classification of body types. He named them **endomorphic, mesomorphic,** and **ectomorphic,** referring to tendencies to be soft and round, square and muscular, or thin and skeletal. Sheldon showed that every body has a blend of these traits in a measurable degree (Figure 6-1).

He devised a complex but reliable formula for labeling body types and recorded them on three seven-point scales. Thus, a completely endomorphic person was scored 7-1-1, a perfect mesomorph 1-7-1, and a total ectomorph 1-1-7. A completely balanced body was rated 4-4-4.

Sheldon claimed that body type is an unalterable inheritance and demonstrated that his system of measurement produced the same scores for people who were tested repeatedly over several years, even after weight changes of as much as 100 pounds.

Other researchers disputed his conviction that body type is a stable trait. In a famous study of malnutrition in which volunteers underwent six months of semi-starvation, scientist Ancel Keys claimed that his subjects had become more ectomorphic. But two years later, they had all returned to their original shapes. This demonstrated most effectively that although shape can be modified, only continued undernutrition will maintain unnatural thinness.

Another scientist, Ethan Allen Sims, overfed volunteers to induce weight gain. His results led to similar conclusions. Weight gain proved hard to achieve and was only temporary. A return to an unforced diet was followed by the loss of the excess weight in almost all of his subjects.

Sheldon went on to describe characteristic temperaments for the various body types he had identified. He repeatedly referred to the endomorph's love of food, often with affection. He wrote of their "deep joy in eating," and observed that for endomorphs, "The soul has its seat in the splendid gut." He showed a refreshing acceptance of both natural and acquired fat by referring to weight gain as "blossoming."

Because Sheldon used complex calculations to determine body type, it is not practical to duplicate his techniques—nor is it necessary. The short questionnaire that follows lists salient characteristics of the three body types (see page 90). The ratio of the total scores is an indicator of the relative strength of the three traits. Note that this questionnaire is but a brief sampling of Sheldon's work. It should not be used for making decisions. It is for illustrative purposes only.

Besides developing his technique for classifying body types, Sheldon and his coworkers studied the natural changes in weight and shape that accompany aging. They discovered that certain body types maintain a stable weight throughout adult life, whereas those people with significant endomorphy gradually fill out until late middle-age, when they are apt to shrink a little (Figure 6-2, p. 91). The amount of normal change is predictable and varies with the degree of endomorphy.

These findings are hardly surprising. They conform precisely with our everyday experience that some people get rounder as they get older, whereas others do not. Only the dictates of fashion and unrealistically dogmatic height and weight charts that make no allowance for age or body type conflict with Sheldon's data. Unfortunately, most people pay more attention to fashion than to physiology and, as a consequence, put themselves in a high risk category for appetite disorders.

BODY TYPE QUESTIONNAIRE

Give yourself one point for every characteristic that is often true. You may check more than one item in a row. Doing so means that you have the attributes of two or more body types.

Endomorphy		*Mesomorphy*		*Ectomorphy*	
Relaxed posture and movement	(✓)	Assertive posture and movement	(●)	Restrained posture and movement	( )
Love of physical comfort	( )	Love of physical adventure	(●)	Secretive emotions, self-consciousness	(✓)
Love of eating	(●)	Love of activity	(●)	Love of quiet	(✓)
Love of social activities	(●)	Pleasure in competition	(●)	Resistance to habit and routine	( )
Love of approval and affection	(●)	Delight in gaining authority	(●)	Slow physical maturation	(✓)
Need for people when troubled	( )	Need for action when troubled	(●)	Need for solitude when troubled	(✓)
Relaxed, friendly with alcohol	( )	Noisy, aggressive when drinking	(●)	Distaste, avoidance of alcohol	(✓)
Soft, rounded physique	( )	Thick, muscular underlayer	(●)	Slender, bony frame	( )
TOTAL ENDOMORPHY	(2)	**TOTAL MESOMORPHY**	(8)	**TOTAL ECTOMORPHY**	( )

Figure 6-2. *Charting weight and age for different body types.*   91

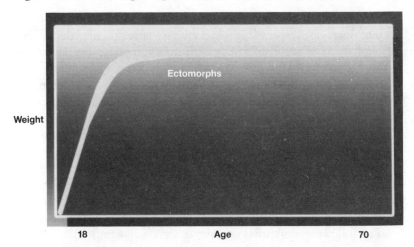

Ectomorphs don't change weight as adults.

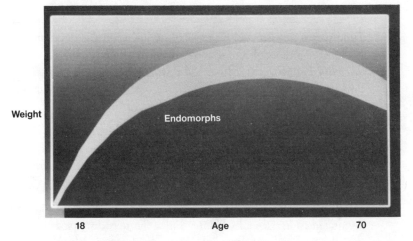

Extreme endomorphs experience much weight change as adults.

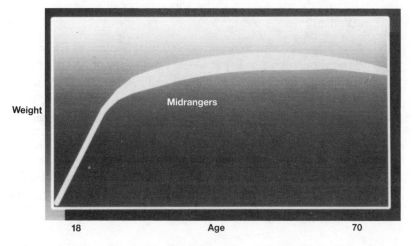

Most of us are midrangers. Our weight and age curve shows moderate change through adult life.

It has been our impression that women with significant meso-morphism are especially vulnerable to appetite disorders. They tend to have squarish frames with an appropriate overlay of fat. Young women with this heritage usually have had an easy time being social and adapting to developmental tasks as children, but they begin to feel uncomfortable about their shape in high school.

They view the need to trim off 15 to 20 pounds as a modest challenge and often confront it by crash dieting. The stubborn resistance their bodies show to being starved comes as a shock to them, and their subsequent development of pathorexic symptoms may be their first experience with failure. Being praised and re-warded for becoming more attractive while they are aware that they are not quite well creates a painful and confusing dilemma. The following story from our files is a good illustration.

June

June was a 16-year-old high school junior when she developed pathorexia. Although she was an excellent student with disciplined study habits, June had distinguished herself most through her athletic prowess. On three varsity teams and captain of the soccer team, she was universally regarded as a leader.

Her consistent patience and good humor resulted in many demands on her time for coaching and supervision. A joy to her parents and an honor student, June seemed to have the world on a string.

Problems began when June decided that it was important that she be invited to her school's Winter Ball. She was dismayed to find that the boys did not act on the hints she dropped. Much to her chagrin, she was faced with the choice of not attending or going with a girlfriend.

June was not about to accept second best. She stayed home, brooded over what had gone wrong, and stared at herself in the mirror in a mood tinged with anger and despair. Suddenly her athlete's body seemed all wrong. Her broad shoulders and muscled calves and thighs were, she decided, the cause of her rejection.

With her customary determination, June immediately set herself a new goal. In three weeks, she lost 15 pounds, putting herself three pounds below the minimum weight for her height, according to a table she found in a women's magazine.

The next shock for June was the discovery that maintaining her new weight was more difficult than achieving it. Her favorite study corner in the kitchen became a place where unmanageable temptations to eat swept over her. While she remained proud of her novel, but barely perceptible, slimness, she was also plagued with sharp mood swings and lost ground in both academics and athletics.

June's parents quickly became involved. Mystified by her upset emotions and then disturbed by her change in behavior, they nevertheless applauded her decision to lose weight because they were perpetually restraining their own appetites. Their first hint that something was seriously amiss came the night they returned home late to find the refrigerator bare of all food and the pantry bereft of bread, cereal, crackers, and cookies. This was the first and worst in a series of solitary raids that June made on the family food supply. These raids resulted in a marked rift with her parents.

June's mother tried a variety of sensible meal plans to help June cope with her cravings, but each failed. After eight weeks of continued pain and tension, June's mother sent her to a dietitian. June's determination to stay underweight was not approved by the dietitian, who recommended more food and referred her to us for psychological help.

June had great difficulty coming to terms with the idea that her muscular body was a characteristic she could not abandon simply because it was no longer fashionable. To accept her figure, she found it necessary to question and revise many other aspects of her identity that she had previously taken for granted. When last we saw her, she had compromised by gaining back between eight and ten of the lost pounds and had settled for an appetite she could control most of the time. She had chosen nutrition for her college major.

Sheldon's work implies that beautiful people with well-balanced physiques are blessed with beautiful genes. Fortunately, we do not have to be "beautiful" to be healthy. For many of us, optimal physical and mental health do not mean that we are necessarily good looking. It is all too likely that our natural allotment of fatty tissues will lie outside the current norms for beauty, both in quantity and distribution.

A NOTE ON HEIGHT AND WEIGHT CHARTS

Almost all height and weight charts published in the popular-press are based on ones the Metropolitan Life Insurance Company produced in 1959 or 1983. There are many variations of these charts, some offering a range of weights for small, medium, and large frames, and others making allowance for clothing weight and heel thickness. The 1983 revision recommends weight a few pounds heavier than the 1959 tables. Both charts recommend weight substantially below the average weight of American adults. No adjustment for age is permitted. The statistician who wrote the original version believed that no one should gain weight after age 25.

The charts are not based on longevity studies, but reflect the experience life insurance companies have with their policies. (Note that the criterion is policies, not customers—a person who has two policies at death gets counted twice!)

There is much professional controversy about the Metropolitan Life tables. Many experts believe they are very misleading. A gerontologist, Dr. Reubin Andres, has produced much more accurate tables that acknowledge that healthy older people are likely to be heavier than they were when they were young. Other tables based on human subjects have been produced. Nevertheless, the Metropolitan tables remain popular—probably because they are simple to understand. We believe that healthy bodies come in all shapes, sizes, and weights. We are leery of attempts to force conformity to standards that do not take the individual into account.

Nevertheless, physical and emotional health is a winning combination, making a striking appearance irrelevant. True happiness is never solely dependent on the shape of our bodies. When an inherently plain person becomes convinced that the route to greater popularity and contentment lies in changing fat distribution through diet programs, the potential for appetite disorders is created.

The vast majority of us inherit proportions that are comfortably within the limits for good health. Occasionally, a genetic predisposition toward unhealthy fatness may occur. At present, our knowledge about this possibility is still limited. We do not know how often such defects appear.

From animal experiments, we know that obesity can be bred into a strain of laboratory mice until all offspring develop the condition, but the chance occurrence of obesity in animals is rare. It is possible that in humans, congenitally determined obesity occurs more often.

Adiposity

The number of fat cells in the body is a second closely related factor in the control of appetite. Normal fat cells are laid down primarily during childhood and adolescence. It is believed that how these cells are formed is determined in part by genetics and in part by nutrition. It is also thought that, by and large, the total number of fat cells cannot be reduced after they have formed, although an unhealthy excess may form during major weight gain.

We conclude from this that feeding patterns in the early years of our lives and in adolescence have a lifelong influence on our shape and, indirectly, on our appetites. If as a child we were indulged with a rich and plentiful supply of food, we may have built up a burden of fat cells that will plague us until we die.

The number of fat cells we possess is not the only variable associated with adiposity. Cell size is also important. The principal purpose of these cells is to be a readily available source of energy for the body. They constitute our fuel supply, and, as such, they are continually being built up or drawn upon. They function by varying in size rather than number.

In healthy people, these variations in size are too subtle to be detectable. Among eating disorder victims, however, this is not so. Because their ineffective appetite control systems cause them to overeat, their fat cells may be subject to major inflation. After reaching a maximum diameter, more cells will form if excess intake continues.

The Guinness Book of World Records has reported on people weighing as much as 1,000 pounds and being crushed by their own weight. Photographs of such people show clearly that their excess weight is in the form of fat. With dieting, those fat cells could be reduced practically to invisibility, but they would not be destroyed, and they would not disappear.

We do not know how much direct effect the size of our fat cells has on our appetite. It is probable that feedback circuits exist that serve to increase hunger as the cells shrink so our energy reserves do not become too depleted. Of course, if we have too many cells to begin with, that alarm system is going to sound too soon, and the struggle to reduce to average weight and then maintain it will be that much more difficult.

There are also indications that the rate of growth of fat cells is related to their size. In other words, the larger they are, the greater is their tendency to further enlarge. To the extent that this is true, it is doubly hard for the overweight person to halt continued weight gain.

Besides the physical effects, excess adiposity has a powerful psychological impact. Sometimes being fat strengthens the resolve to lose weight, but all too often it fosters a depressed mood that typically leads to overeating and more weight gain.

Whether an internal monitoring function exists or whether fat cells have only a psychological effect on appetite, their presence in excess creates a form of obesity that is especially resistant to weight reduction programs. The condition is most common in people who become heavy in childhood or adolescence. Many such endomorphic people are quite at home with their soft, round physiques, and they enjoy temperaments that match their appearance. Research indicates that their mental health and self-respect fall within normal limits, and they live full and happy lives. They never expect to be slim, and they have always been aware that their above-average weight can inflate into obesity when they give in to their overactive appetites.

Others, however, never accept their bodies. They fight a constant battle with themselves, and their sense of well-being is inversely proportional to their weight.

Given the public's preoccupation with weight loss and with slenderness as a hallmark of beauty, it is easy to understand their unhappiness. Heavy people do not need our sympathy, but they do need our support. Thoughtless remarks and discrimination are common experiences. Perhaps the expression "She has such a pretty face . . . ," is the one phrase most often uttered by well meaning but misinformed people.

Laura

Early photographs of Laura suggest that she probably was regarded as a "pleasantly plump" baby. By the age of five, however, she was a typical little girl complete with skinny legs and knobby knees.

She has early memories of her mother telling her, after she had had enough to eat, that she must be careful not to end up looking like Aunt Susan (Mother's overweight sister), whom Mother never failed to ridicule. Laura remembers leaving the table hungry, but receiving praise when she mentioned not having satisfied her appetite.

During Laura's preteen and teenage years, her mother and father commented daily on her adorable and sweet appearance. When Laura showed interest in what her folks considered to be extra food, her parents always told her not to ruin her figure and complexion. Dad would then suggest that "his ladies go on a little shopping spree." The family was well off financially, and buying new outfits was a well-established female role, second only to cooking and laundering.

*Laura recalls **always** feeling a bit hungry but feeling very beautiful and refined in her expensive clothes. She would, in fact, binge on clothing, often buying outfits she had no use for but that she thought looked good on her. Today, many of them remain unworn in her closet.*

At 25, Laura married and within a few months became pregnant. Knowledge of her impending weight gain seemed to give Laura permission to eat, and eat she did. Before the first trimester was over, her physician expressed concern about her excessive weight gain. Laura denied the seriousness of this warning and continued to eat all she wanted of everything. The weight gain continued, the warnings continued, the ignoring continued. Finally, Laura developed toxemia, and the delivery of her baby had to be induced one month early.

Following the birth of her child, Laura was able to shed only five of the 65 pounds she had gained. In reviewing her case history, it appears that a foundation of extra adipose cells developed during infancy and remained dormant because of Laura's strict restraint of food intake until she became pregnant. Once she gave up controlling her appetite, the weight gain was rapid.

Laura has remained at least 40 pounds over her prepregnancy weight, and though she is not happy with her appearance, there have been no further medical complications.

As we might reasonably expect, the digestive system and the brain each have a large role in controlling appetite and eating. Sensory organs in the stomach, the intestine, and the liver monitor the system's current need for food and help regulate eating behavior on an hour-to-hour basis.

The brain's role is probably more tuned toward long-term maintenance of the whole organism, deciding when there is a need to increase or decrease fat stores. The brain is possibly a nutritional

Metabolism and Appetite

victims

monitor also, subtly directing us to consume needed quantities of protein, vitamins, and minerals to maintain optimal health and functioning.

The stomach swells and shrinks in the course of its work and secretes various gastric juices during that cycle. Normal individuals seem able to sense these and other physiological variations, such as blood sugar level, and are able to translate them into the discomfort of hunger and the pleasure of satiety. It is likely that healthy persons pick up these subtle cues and the obvious, more visual ones—like the amount of food that has disappeared from the plate—and stop eating to avoid the unpleasant consequences of overindulgence.

Anorexics, bulimics, and compulsive eaters seem to lack this ability. Experiments have shown that their experience of hunger has less connection with the amount of food present in their stomachs than is the case with normal persons. Anorexics feel bloated when very small amounts of food enter the stomach. Bulimics and compulsive eaters may continue eating even though their stomachs are full. Conversely, both anorexics and bulimics fail to recognize their need for food and, in its absence, can go for much longer periods of time than normal people without feeling hungry.

Unfortunately, for bulimics this attribute is more than cancelled out by their inability to refrain from eating when food is present. Experiments have shown them to be significantly more aware of and aroused by the sight or smell of food. A physiological reason for this has been shown to be their tendency to secrete the digestive hormone **insulin** when they see, smell, or think about attractive foods. Insulin, which is needed for absorption of food, triggers the appetite, and excess insulin not only arouses the appetite but also maintains it when the stomach is full. This leads many pathorexic people to continue eating even though they feel physically uncomfortable and know they would be wise to stop.

This phenomenon has been measured by comparing the response to sugar of eating disordered patients with people with normal appetites. Healthy people tire of the taste of sugar as their stomachs fill, but pathorexics are happy to continue eating sweets and desserts for much longer periods of time. These differences go a long way to explain the familiar conflict between appetite and willpower that people with appetite disorders experience each time they have more food available than they need.

The hormone imbalances that are associated with too much insulin are complex and vary greatly among individuals. They also have widely varying effects on energy, mood, hunger, and other physical sensations. The craving for food late at night, for example, may well be triggered physiologically. So, too, may be desires for unusual foods, loss of ability to concentrate, mood swings, sweating, dizziness, and other minor upsets. The relationships between nutrition and a sense of well-being are only just being unraveled.

An unresolved question about hyperinsulinism, as this condition is called, concerns the extent to which it may be induced by dieting. It is well known that the body reacts defensively to sharp reductions in food supply. Metabolism slows down, tissue replacement is deferred, and both fat and lean mass is sacrificed. To promote eating behavior, the appetite may quicken.

When dieters refeed, their bodies rebuild fat stores first and often compensate for the trauma of dieting by laying down more fat than was lost. This explains the common dilemma of quick weight loss being followed by a regain of weight to a new and higher total weight. Hyperinsulinism is the body's response to unhealthy weight loss and may intensify with each round of dieting and weight gain.

Our experience indicates that for some people a quick loss of as little as six pounds may trigger pathorexia. Thus, the treadmill of chronic dieting and perpetual hunger in the presence of food can begin with the seemingly innocent first step of trimming a few pounds for cosmetic effect.

Appetite and the Brain

The brain's role in controlling appetite can be considered under two categories: instinctual behaviors that happen without thought and psychological behaviors that cause us to act according to how we feel or how we believe we must feel. It is the former that we discuss in this section. Psychological factors are considered in the next chapter.

The part of the brain that influences appetite seems to be located near the **hypothalamus,** which is a primitive organ that we share with much older and less evolved animals, including reptiles and fish. It is here that the mechanism that triggers insulin release is located. Because of the limitations on experimenting with live humans, much of our knowledge of hypothalamic appetite control is derived from work with animals, especially rats and mice.

It has been found that this nerve center is very important to rodents and exerts major control over their appetite and adiposity. Normal adult rats generally maintain their weight within close limits. That weight is called their **setpoint.** When, however, tiny cuts are made in areas of the brain close to the hypothalamus, the animals make drastic changes in their diets. Depending on the locations of these lesions, they may gain weight or lose it.

After a certain amount of weight change has occurred, the rats actively work to maintain their new size. They counteract, to the

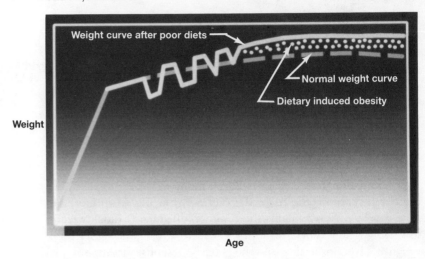

Figure 6-3. *The more dieting a person does, the greater is the rise in setpoint.*

extent they can, any forced feeding or fasting their experimenters impose upon them. Rats that have become obese seek to stay fat. Rats with depleted fat stores resist attempts to restore them to a more healthy weight. The brain lesions have altered their setpoints.

The implications of this research for humans are still being explored, but it raises some interesting speculations. It is possible, for example, that normal weight, although genetically determined in part, may also be governed by mechanisms in the brain that could sometimes operate without regard to overall health.

Healthy humans apparently have a clearly defined setpoint. Unlike rats, however, the human setpoint varies. First, for all but the most ectomorphic persons, setpoint rises steadily through middle age, and then tends to fall again (see Figure 6-2, p. 93). Second, setpoint varies with the amount of physical energy a person customarily exerts. Active bodies that would be hampered by the need to move heavy fat stores carry less fat. Sedentary people can have more fat stores, which have survival value during famine, sickness, and childbirth.

The logic of survival (which has nothing to do with fashion) dictates that bodies subject to frequent deprivation will do better if they have higher setpoints, and thus more fat stores. This vital mechanism causes the minor tragedy of **dietary induced obesity.** The more often fat people diet, the higher their setpoints rise. The effect is shown graphically in Figure 6-3 above. It is shown more dramatically in the memberships of weight loss clinics and clubs, where the same faces (and bodies) recycle after reaching a new setpoint. Ironically, the clinics that induce the fastest weight loss also cause the greatest rise in setpoint, and thus the fastest regain of weight.

An excellent discussion of this subject can be found in the book *The Dieter's Dilemma,* which is listed in the suggested readings at the end of this book.

Some anorexics have brain dysfunctions that sharply reduce their appetites. Indirect evidence suggests that some types of physical abnormalities contribute to some forms of appetite disorder. It is possible that severe emotional distress causes hormonal imbalances that in turn cause appetite and weight loss.

Certain drugs that alter brain chemistry provoke and inhibit appetite and cause temporary weight changes. This raises the distinct possibility that medications may be developed that can alter appetite and restore normal eating patterns.

Although the hypothalamus plays a major part in appetite control, it has a far less significant role in humans than in rats and other experimental animals. The human brain is dominated by a massive **cerebral cortex** that other animals lack. The cortex is our cognitive center. It is where we store information and learn to make decisions based on knowledge rather than instinct. Our cortex gives us the power to interfere, modify, and override many of the instinctual patterns of the lower brain centers. In the long run, what we **learn** to do has more influence on our behavior than what we are born **able** to do. It is most important to always remember that no matter how deeply enmeshed in an eating disorder a person may be, the road to recovery still lies chiefly in learning new ways to look at life, ways that allow for growth and understanding.

Another way that the brain contributes to eating disorders is by creating a sense of calm during bingeing or after vomiting by releasing the body's natural pain killers, called **endorphins.** Endorphins are chemically related to morphine and are potent pain killers. They are released whenever the body is placed under severe stress, such as injury or excessive exercise. The runner's high, a feeling of well-being experienced by athletes, is an example of endorphin release. Unfortunately, like morphine and heroin, endorphins can create an addiction. Bulimarexics become as addicted to purging as narcotic addicts are to heroin.

Studies show raised endorphin levels following bingeing in obese subjects and vomiting in bulimics, just as they have been detected after other physical stresses have been imposed on the subject. We close this chapter with a case history that illustrates the phenomenon of auto-addiction.

Pam

Pam was a patient we treated on and off for two years. She returned after six months without therapy, saying that although her life had improved dramatically and she no longer felt prompted to binge and purge because of stress, she had experienced an irresistible urge to resume vomiting. Discussion led us to conclude that Pam had become addicted to the feeling of calm that followed the purge, a calm that she said was just like the runner's high she used to experience when she ran several miles a day. She noted, too, that purging had replaced exercise in her life, a change that puzzled and troubled her. By recognizing that her addiction had shifted from a psychological to a physiological pressure, Pam had the strength to reduce the frequency of her purges, although she continues to find them a source of tranquility that she calls on from time to time.

SUMMARY

The major physical factors that affect appetite and eating disorders are heredity, adiposity, metabolism, and brain functions. They all interact and are closely linked.

Much of a person's size, shape, coloring, and personality is closely determined by genetic inheritance, with 50 percent contributed by each parent. Children of obese parents have an 80 percent chance of being heavy, regardless of whether they are raised by biological or foster parents. Similarly, muscularity and slenderness are inherited traits. Every person has a unique blend of inherited characteristics.

Because the healthy range of normal adiposity is far greater than current fashion regards as attractive, heavy people feel much pressure to reduce. It is an avoidable tragedy that the more unsuccessful dieting they do the higher their ultimate weight is likely to be.

Eating and appetite disorders occur when determined attempts are made to alter inherited body type and established adiposity.

The mechanisms that govern eating behaviors consist of digestive and cerebral (brain) components working together. The digestive tract, from mouth to colon, is a delicately balanced system for processing food and signaling nutritional needs. Food abuse can disrupt this system, creating appetite when there is no need for more food in the stomach, or satiety and bloated feelings even when a person is starving.

Appetite centers in the brain are located near the hypothalamus. These centers seem to control long-term trends in nutrition and weight; they also aid in arousing and suppressing appetite. The function of these centers is also affected by food abuse and dieting. Chronic dieting, for example, is interpreted by the brain as a shortage of available food. In response, the brain is likely to raise the body's setpoint so that more fat can be stored.

The brain also controls the secretion of the body's natural painkillers, called endorphins. Food abuse and purging can cause this system to overreact, reinforcing behaviors that release more endorphins, and encouraging pathology rather than recovery.

CHAPTER REVIEW

◆ ─────────────── VOCABULARY ─────────────── ◆

cerebral cortex   the largest part of the human brain; the center in which conscious decisions are made. The cerebral cortex can override impulses and instincts prompted by more primitive parts of the brain.

endocrine   type of gland which secretes substances (hormones) inside the body.

heredity   the passage of inherited characteristics through genes from parents to children.

hormones   complex chemicals secreted by the body that control many biological functions.

hypothalamus   a part of the brain, close to the top of the spinal column, associated with appetite and other automatic behaviors.

metabolism   the processes by which food, water, and air sustain a living organism.

setpoint   the weight a person or animal maintains and returns to after dieting or overfeeding. Setpoint varies with age and activity levels, and may be raised if the organism is subject to chronic deprivation.

◆ ─────────── FOR YOUR CONSIDERATION ─────────── ◆

◆ Bodies come in all sizes and shapes, but fashion finds only narrow ranges acceptable for women, and also, to a lesser extent, for men.

◆ To be counted "just right," a woman needs to be below average weight and above average height! Clearly only a few can qualify. Why do you think that nature breeds so much diversity, while fashion demands conformity, and rewards scarcity?

◆ Review Sheldon's body types. Can you fit yourself and your parents into his model? What significance does your body type have on your sense of personal identity?

◆ William Sheldon was highly respected during his lifetime, but largely ignored after he died in 1976. Why do you think this may have happened?

Distribution of weight

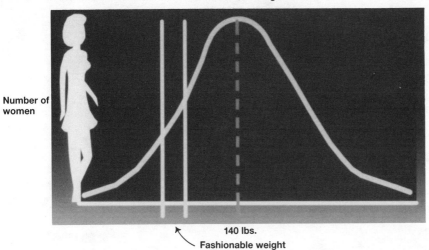

Number of women

140 lbs.
Fashionable weight

Distribution of height

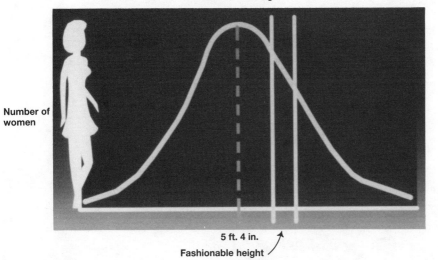

Number of women

5 ft. 4 in.
Fashionable height

THE PSYCHOLOGY OF EATING DISORDERS

This chapter will help you:

1. Learn how contemporary social norms and values cause eating disorders.
2. See that eating disorders stem from a search for personal identity, a need to reduce stress, a fear of growing up, a history of abuse in childhood, and other psychiatric problems.
3. Understand how healthy attempts to be disciplined can turn into serious problems with food.

◆

*"Every time Jack worked
late at the office, I'd empty
the refrigerator and then
head for the bathroom."*

Human beings, like all living organisms, seek food spontaneously and respond physically to the sight or smell of food. Unlike other organisms, however, humans do not have simple, inborn characteristics that set limits to that search and response.

As soon as we are born, our parents and other caretakers move to socialize our food-seeking behavior. In the process, they distort the relationship between our nutritional needs and our appetite.

THE BIRTH OF FOOD-SEEKING BEHAVIOR

In the beginning, this is all done for our own good, of course. The process gets under way the first time our mother offers us affection instead of food when we are hungry. From then on the interference never ends. First comes the scheduling of meals to meet the needs of the family. Later there is encouragement to eat all the food prepared. Then there is good food versus poor food, treats and luxuries, the starving children in Asia, feasts, stories of famines, waiting until everyone is served, never taking the biggest slice, permissible snacks and forbidden snacks, watching one's weight, and getting a good breakfast every morning.

There is guidance and manipulation. There are good examples and bad examples. There is education, and there is propaganda.

The only thing there never is, is silence.

Although most of our attitudes toward food and eating are formed in childhood, some major changes may occur at the second threshhold of life, entry to adulthood. This is a time when the influence of peers may shift behavior away from established family patterns. Also at this time, working parents and busy schedules often crowd out regular meals altogether.

A process that has been called "grazing" is substituted for breakfast, lunch, and dinner. Convenience foods—prepackaged snacks, fast foods, candy, and microwaved leftovers—are eaten at will throughout the day. The connection between appetite and nutrition is lost. There is no structured family time.

A common behavior that occurs at this time is learning to vomit to avoid the consequences of overindulgence in alcohol.

College students living in dormitories often have to deal with dining hall rules that encourage food abuse. Bingeing, hoarding, and stealing often begin as ways to cope with rushed meals, kitchens closing early, and inadequate quantities of quality food. Poorly prepared food can lead to reliance on candy or desserts to compensate for inedible cafeteria meals. Weight gain from too much starchy food may lead to imprudent dieting and self-starvation.

Young people who move into their own living quarters and cook for themselves for the first time also have a tendency to take short cuts with food preparation. In a susceptible individual, these changes can set in motion a drift into eating disorders.

These processes are both social and psychological. The social components are the inputs from family and society to the individual and the responses of the individual. The psychological components are the interactions between the individual's genetic endowment and those parental and social inputs.

The prospect of ever truly disentangling the genetic from the social inputs so that the unique contribution of each can be identified is remote, but we do know that constitutional (that is, genetic) differences affect what we learn and how we respond.

Inherent psychological variables surely cause some people to favor the parental injunction to "eat what is served" over the conflicting injunction "don't gain weight." Others will adopt the reverse position. Also, the degree to which the stomach and the brain affect behavior in the face of social attempts to override these injunctions varies from person to person.

So each one of us grows up in a unique confusion of conflicting and contradictory messages about the primary sustaining force in life—our appetite.

Because of the physical necessity that we eat every few hours, it is likely that no aspect of our growth and maturation receives as much attention as our eating patterns. We are taught to associate food with a host of connected attitudes and values, some of which are clearly detrimental to our health.

For example, most of us learn to appreciate the taste of candy, which is nutritionally poor but frequently associated with affection, and to recoil from nourishing vegetables because they are so often presented with coercion. In early childhood, we develop a hierarchy of preference for various foods, and our parents find it difficult to resist the temptation to control our behavior by offering and withdrawing favored goodies.

The relationship between flavor and appetite is fascinating. We are learning rapidly, but still have far to go. Flavor is the most intimate environmental factor affecting appetite and probably has important consequences for health. We know that humans and animals have a powerful tendency to prefer sweet, and therefore ripe, fruits and vegetables; this mechanism has obvious survival value.

A Taste for Sugar and Fats

The relatively recent development (that is, since the Industrial Revolution) of techniques for the inexpensive refining and manufacture of sugar has led to the growth of huge companies dedicated to its production and has greatly increased the sweetness of our diets. Human biology has not changed to compensate for this environmental revolution. We still prefer sweet food, though this preference is likely to be more hazardous than healthy.

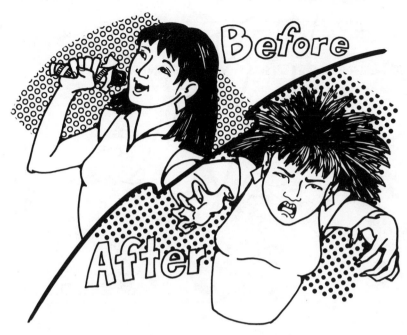

Figure 7-1. *Sugar can have monstrous effects on many of us. Do you know how sugar affects you?*

Some people sense that their personalities change dramatically, and for the worse, when they consume sugar (Figure 7-1, p. 110). A patient told us this:

> "*When I get into sugars, I'm a Jekyll and Hyde. I numb out. I'm totally out of touch with my feelings, but I'll rationalize anything to keep eating. I'll even think I need to gain weight! I can see it in my mother, too. When she's on sugar, I can't trust her with information. She twists and distorts anything I say.*"

A similar situation exists with respect to fats. These cheap, high-calorie substances have little flavor themselves, but when they are added to other foods, they greatly enhance their palatability. Because they are relatively inexpensive, they are used in vast quantities by the food industry.

Many experts think these changes have caused a massive deformation in the world's nutrition. Others find no reason for concern. As we await hard information, it is wise to monitor and restrain our personal consumption of sugar, sweeteners, and fats, and we should seek to rediscover the subtler flavors of less processed foods.

A NOTE ON NONNUTRITIVE SWEETENERS

Sugar substitutes were originally marketed when sugar was scarce or temporarily expensive. Now they are mainly used to reduce the caloric content of foods, especially in soft drinks. Because they are organic chemicals used in relatively high concentrations, there is constant concern about their safety. There is much less concern about their effect on appetite and food intake, but some recent research and our clinical impressions suggest that nonnutritive sweeteners stimulate the appetite so that the total caloric content of meals that include them matches or exceeds the calories consumed in meals where sugar is used. We also suspect that drinking diet soda between meals acts as a powerful appetite stimulant that results in more food consumption rather than less.

The Link Between Eating and Affection

The net result of this barrage of manipulation—familial, social, and commercial—is to create for each of us an artificial structure of needs and motivations when dealing with food and eating.

Although every one of us is different, however, some trends and tendencies can be applied to all. Surely the most widespread characteristic is the link between eating and affection. It is a simple human pleasure to feed those we love. When our own search for love is inhibited, many of us find comfort by substituting food just as, if our search for food were frustrated, we would surely find comfort in the closeness and warmth of love.

Psychoanalysts have developed comprehensive explanations of human behavior based on the interaction between affection and feeding in the first months of a baby's life. Anyone who has spent time with weight control programs is aware that, while almost all food is hard to resist, Grandma's cake and Mom's apple pie are the treats that are most difficult to refuse. The psychology of infancy finds an echo and a re-enactment in every decade of our lives.

It may be that people who experience much uncertainty or insecurity as children are especially susceptible to appetite disorders. Animal studies have shown that unpredictable feeding schedules create increased appetites in young rats, and there is clinical evidence suggesting parallels with children from troubled families.

Beth

Beth was a 16-year-old only child whose parents were divorced. Both parents had remarried and had joint custody of their daughter. After several months of treatment, Beth came to recognize that she felt responsible for keeping all four parents and stepparents happy. The stress generated by this impossible responsibility precipitated her illness. Beth felt that the concern generated by the illness kept her stepfamilies cooperating, and it also allowed her to avenge the hurt she felt when her parents divorced. Later, she realized that her folks had made many problems worse because, although they worried about her, they blamed each other for the situation.

Beth gradually separated herself from her parents' conflicting expectations. Counseling helped her to recognize that her anger was misplaced. As the stress eased, her bulimia subsided. As her health improved, her parents no longer needed to be in such close contact with each other. The vicious cycle of conflicts that had reinforced the symptoms was reversed. When the pressure was relieved, Beth learned how to appreciate her extended family instead of feeling oppressed by it.

Anxiety, Depression, and Eating Disorders

Perhaps the most compelling impulse to abuse food stems from anxiety. Fear, insecurity, and uneasiness that have no obvious source create an unpleasant state of tension we call anxiety. Periods of transition—from home to school, childhood to adolescence, and adolescence to adulthood, to name just three we all experience—are times of heightened anxiety. In every person's life there are many others.

One way to reduce anxiety is turning to behaviors that we know make us feel better and more secure. The most universal and the most reliable of these is eating. From the first day of our lives, we have found comfort in food. No wonder our paths through the turmoils of adolescence pass repeatedly through the doors of fast food outlets! When stress is severe and chronic, when it seems that no one understands us, the pantry, the refrigerator, and the convenience store offer tempting temporary relief.

When the fear of weight gain compounds anxiety, tranquility from eating is compromised. Adopting purging to compensate for eating is a logical, but hazardous, step toward a solution far worse than the problem. As we learned in Chapter 6, purging provides its own perverse rewards. The binge and purge cycle initially relieves a lot of anxiety. But it also creates a whole new set of problems which raise anxiety once more. A bulimic spiral may be the unhappy consequence of attempting to cope alone with stresses that require the help of family, friends, and perhaps professional counselors.

In Chapter 3 we discussed appetite changes that accompany depression, and we suggested that bulimia may be a symptom of severe depressive illness. Feeling depressed—sad, lonely, lost, and without energy—is also an aspect of everyday life, for all of us. When depression is associated with an identifiable event and is short-lived, it is not abnormal, but such depression may also be associated with food abuse for the same reasons that anxiety is. Food is a reliable source of comfort and warmth, a source that can be tapped without having to ask other people for help and without having to expose our unhappiness to others or to risk their rejection. Just as with anxiety, the chronic use of food to relieve depression can lead to food abuse, further isolation, and increased depression.

Child Abuse and Eating Disorders

A special case of extreme stress that young people are exposed to is sexual and emotional abuse. Such abuse is particularly likely to give rise to eating disorders, along with other psychological and physical problems.

Sexual abuse occurs whenever a person with superior power, authority, or strength coerces another to share or provide any kind of sexual intimacy whatsoever. It is estimated that one in four girls and one in seven boys experience sexual abuse before they are eighteen.

Sexual abuse traumatizes victims. It destroys trust when it is perpetrated by a friend, relative, or neighbor, as is usually the case. It damages or destroys normal sources of pleasure and affection by associating them with pain and fear. And all too often it cripples family supports when it is kept secret, or the victim's feelings of outrage and violation are not acknowledged or addressed.

Emotional abuse includes every form of irresponsible child care short of physical assault. It ranges from neglect to overprotection, and from idealization to contempt. When it is sustained, it is inevitably psychologically injurious. It frequently causes eating disorders.

Abused children who do not get the help they need live in a twilight world. They feel anxious, depressed, oppressed, helpless, hopeless, and worthless. It is no wonder that many, perhaps most of them, turn back to food for comfort, and then develop eating disorders. Certain emotional abuses are predictably followed by specific forms of pathorexia. Neglect is often a precursor to bulimia. Neurotic overinvolvement by parents leads to anorexia. When the abuse is deliberate or malevolent, the disorders are likely to be severe and life-threatening. Often, the rejection of nurturance that is a central aspect of anorexia and the cycles of ingestion and expulsion in bulimia act out in symbolic fashion feelings of loss and rage that cannot be expressed openly; we explain this psychological substitution more fully next.

One important human attribute is our ability to find substitute satisfactions when our primary needs cannot be met. Most of these compensatory mechanisms work to our advantage; for example, when a child who loses a parent succeeds in bonding with another supportive adult. Sometimes, however, these substitutions are symbolic instead of real. The analogy between sports and warfare is a commonly recognized and approved transformation.

Looking for Substitutions ✓

Occasionally substitution works against us. Clinical psychologists often find that an emotional disorder becomes more difficult to treat when it is forbidden or when inhibited thoughts or behaviors are acted out through acceptable but inappropriate symbolic gestures.

The acts of eating, fasting, and vomiting can easily become symbols of affection, control, and anger. If these emotional associations are powerful and compelling and the same emotions do not have a normal outlet in daily life, the symbolic acts may become addictive behaviors. Because these behaviors are only symbolic, they never truly work to resolve problems. Nevertheless, they do provide a modest sense of relief and, as such, get repeated over and over in a fruitless quest for peace.

Anorexics are especially prone to entrapment in these fantasies. Eating and fat become symbols of weakness, whereas fasting is equated with power.

While well on the way to recovery from bulimarexia, one young woman had a relapse into anorexia when she fell in love. Believing that she had to avoid being "just another ordinary person," she became convinced that she would be able to stop her boyfriend from leaving if she quit eating lunch.

Another anorexic who was having romantic difficulties invited her boyfriend to dinner with the family. When he was late in arriving, she turned to her mother and said coolly, "If he doesn't come, I'm not eating this food!"

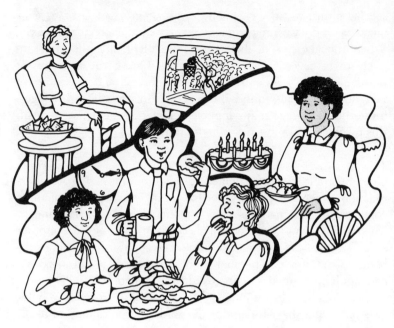

Figure 7-2. *Eating and food have become integral parts of our social activities.*

The Effect of Social Pressures

Another almost universal custom is the inclusion of food in ceremonies of celebration (Figure 7-2). Most of us feel a strong desire to use food to enhance any pleasurable occasion. Although Thanksgiving dinner has a clear historical connection with the harvest, other everyday situations have become inappropriately food-related: football on television prompts us to break out beer and pretzels; movies are not the same without popcorn; a coffee break tends to be enriched with a doughnut.

These and many similar situations can infiltrate our lives to the point where we no longer regard the associated foods as treats but as essential accompaniments to the occasions. Without them, the events would no longer be enjoyable. When food consumption becomes linked in this way to between-meal activities, the influence of physical cues that signal satisfaction are diminished. Our appetites get triggered by our environment instead of our bodies.

A widespread but hazardous behavior pattern is the willingness to let other people decide for us what and how much we should eat. As a mark of respect to a host, we naturally try to eat what is offered for a meal or refreshment. Meanwhile our host, out of respect for us, tries to serve enough food to make sure no one remains hungry. All too often the net result is that significant overfeeding takes place. This often sets a standard for subsequent socializing.

In addition, 20th century abundance has created a situation in which many families prepare, daily, as lavish a table as in the past would have been reserved for feasts. The consequence is that most of us have established a level of richness and quantity in food service that far exceeds what is needed for good health.

For many people, affluence has led to the assumption that hunger can and should be banished. Indeed, there are people who cannot remember when they last felt hungry. From there it is a short step to becoming afraid of being hungry. Such people embrace overeating and perhaps other forms of pathorexia as their salvation from the normal, invigorating experience of hunger that is a thrice daily event for healthy persons.

The common thread through these examples of the social pressures to alter our eating behaviors is that they all serve to separate our appetites from our nutritional needs. (Indeed, this is often a conscious goal: the host who can overcome a guest's reluctance to accept a second helping scores a social victory.) In this way our appetites are redirected, and we lose touch with our personal needs while learning to substitute social customs. This often leads to excessive eating, obesity, an unfashionable appearance, and the disapproval of the very persons who previously encouraged the overindulgence.

Girls and women seem especially vulnerable to this cruel irony because they are raised to be sensitive to the needs of others. As children, they allow themselves to be overfed in order to conform to parental wishes, only to discover as teenagers that they are criticized for being fat.

Many women diet themselves thin as they search for a husband and marry at the lightest weight of their adult lives. Only later do they permit their natural size and shape to emerge. Being unnaturally thin during courtship creates unreasonable expectations about appearance that can cause unnecessary stress after marriage. Such women (and their husbands) are victims of a double bind in which the aesthetic values that bring them together are abandoned once they are committed in marriage.

A similar dilemma occurs at mealtimes in families that stress both companionship at meals and conformity to fashion (Figure 7-3). Two contradictory messages are sent: "Come eat with us," and "Be slim and lovely."

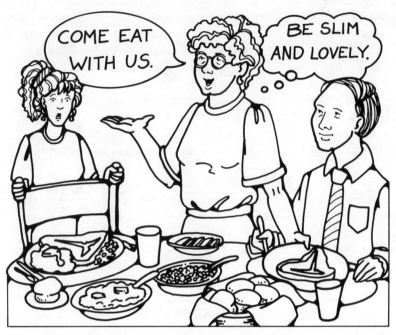

Figure 7-3. *Our families and friends may expect companion-ship at meals while also requiring conformity to fashion (be slim and lovely).*

This conflict always causes a loss of self-respect for persons programmed to please others. The misery is particularly intense in adolescence if there is a significant failure to arouse the interest of potential lovers. Since making friends and attracting sexual partners is a hugely important aspect of life for young adults, some of them find themselves totally consumed with this project.

Again, women are especially prone to problems because they know that their appearance is a vital part of the dating game and a major aspect of their sense of personal identity. If they lack social confidence, they often blame their figures for their disappointments, ignoring the fact that many of their equally imperfect peers pair off with ease. The binge and purge syndrome often develops as a consequence of this crisis. Initially, the victim experiences it as a blessed relief from the pressures of the double bind—being able to eat all that is served, yet still maintaining or losing weight.

But the cycle of overeating and vomiting induces its own varieties of psychic pain. Victims soon feel alone and trapped in a disgusting but inescapable behavior pattern that takes over their lives. A facade of contentment often conceals an inner suicidal despair. Now, when a chance for sexual relations occurs, the eating-disordered woman is likely to sabotage it, or to pursue it mechanically and lovelessly. She may choose an uncaring partner because a sense of unworthiness pervades her whole personality. Bulimarexia is a vicious and punishing emotional disorder.

Judy

Judy came to see us at age 20 for help with a very severe case of bulimarexia. She had been diagnosed as anorexic in high school and had seen several therapists, although she had never been hospitalized. She reported years of "cold war" with her father, who was a graduate of a prestigious Eastern business school. The cold war usually took the form of her father being disappointed, and Judy usually retreated to her mother in the kitchen. She and her mother shared quiet criticisms of her dad, but neither ever spoke up to him.

Judy continued to see her parents regularly even after she moved out of the house. She reported still feeling like an object to them, being walked around and "shown" to people at cocktail parties and other social occasions. Typically, her folks would describe how Judy was going to put herself through law school by doing television commercials. "She's so pretty, she already has offers," they would exaggerate.

Even though she recognized her nonperson status in their eyes, Judy would say, "But what right do I have to get angry with them? They are my parents and they really only want what's best for me. My father doesn't mean to be harsh. He just wants to see me live up to my full potential." Meanwhile the secret bingeing and vomiting continued.

*Judy gradually improved. First she had to realize how unrealistic her parents' goals for her were. Then she had to realize that she had a right to set her **own** goals—to decide what she wanted for herself. Eventually, she was vomiting only once or twice a week. At this point, she decided to move far away and change her career. This broke her dependency on her father's opinions and allowed Judy to set herself free. When we last heard from her, she was doing well and felt truly happy for the first time she could remember. Her relationship with her parents was still difficult, but Judy was reconciled to its being somewhat forced until they became accustomed to her emancipation.*

Another young woman who maintained a weight of 100 pounds by starving and then bingeing and purging wrote this letter:

"I'm mad at Mike (her husband). I'm mad because sexually I **can** *taunt him now. When my weight was 'healthy'—your word—he wasn't interested in sex. Now I hurt, and this is how he likes me.* **Now** *he wants me.*

"I remember his mother's saying—after I had been bulimic for a long time, and she knew it—'What is bulimia but a bit of vomit in the toilet.' And I think Mike feels the same.

"Maybe I'm blowing it up way out of proportion and it isn't that important, but it **is** *an hour of eating and the same amount of time vomiting in a steaming hot bathroom just to keep warm. It is an hour of crying while at the same time getting sick. It is more time wondering if I've gotten everything up, and if I am going to gain weight from it. It is almost intolerable amounts of loneliness, guilt, shame, and fear. It is time I could use doing things I love to do.*

"Mike's mom said she thought I was a 'lady'—that I would make Mike a good 'executive's wife.' How is what I do in any way 'ladylike?' It doesn't seem to matter how much I hurt, so long as I keep up the mask.

*"At least I understand now a little bit about why it is important to me that I be small—***it is my power.*** It is a vicious circle— this mask I hate that I have to keep, and the longer I keep it, the more I hate it; but also the more necessary it becomes. For this mask-lady-executive wife,* **taunting** *is what makes me bite back my opinions, or even share myself the way I always dreamed I would with my own husband. It keeps me from hating him for what I do—in part because this is how he 'wants' me! It is a* **Beauty and the Beast** *story—and I play both parts."*

DIETING AND DENIAL

The common trigger for all eating disorders is dieting. A mechanism that makes them chronic is denial. The illusion develops that being thinner, eating less, renouncing food, or burning up all fat deposits will resolve emotional distress. Denial prevents the victim from realizing that no problems are being solved, although others are being created.

As a modest exercise in self-discipline, going on a diet can be a real plus. Everyone feels better for being in control, and losing a few pounds or an inch around the waist may be America's favorite pastime. The extra self-confidence gained from giving up desserts, for example, couples a psychological boost with some physical benefits.

The increased well-being that follows brief dieting often helps dieters put a bad experience behind them, or make a start on a new project. With that accomplished, a return to normal eating patterns follows for most people. Eating disorders develop when this sequence fails to occur.

Some people delude themselves by thinking that if a little weight loss feels good, more will feel better. Related illusions that grow from this idea are that fasting is noble, eating is a sign of weakness, fat is dirty, and elimination of fat from the body is possible and a worthy goal.

Once these irrational ideas gain a foothold, a serious eating disorder is virtually ensured. The disorder develops because the person's mind and body become adversaries. First the mind decides to renounce food. This usually causes the body to increase appetite. Eventually the craving to eat becomes irresistible, and instead of eating a little, the person binges. This creates guilt, which is answered with a redoubled determination to fast. A vicious cycle is quickly established (Figure 7-4, p. 120).

For people who lack enough respect for their bodies to avoid abusing them, or whose competitive instinct dominates their good sense, the cycle of bingeing and starving gets punctuated with purging and excessive exercise.

The cycle of deprivation, appetite increase, binge, guilt, purge, and redeprivation can easily become a major feature of a person's life. Soon the shame and secrecy it engenders further isolate the victim. Once that happens, bulimia is all the person knows.

Dieting

"Why do people fight so hard to stay ill?" one nurse asked. The answer is that denial is part of the illness. Just as with alcoholics, helping eating disordered individuals to admit they are ill is a first major step toward recovery. And also, as is true of alcoholics, family members of the eating-disordered will deny and delay acknowledging the disease, often until serious illness has been established.

Denial is a defense mechanism that was identified by Sigmund Freud at the turn of the century. Freud believed that mentally ill individuals hid their true feelings by mostly unconscious use of defense mechanisms. Reality was too harsh for these frail or trau-

Denial

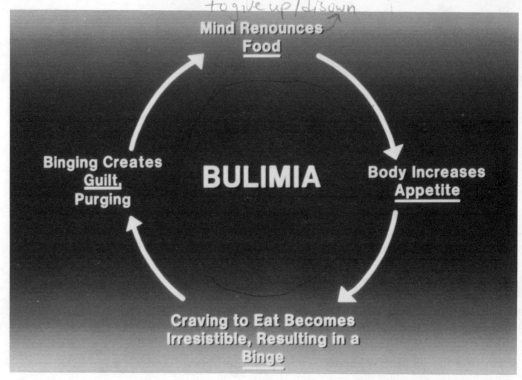

to give up/disown

Mind Renounces Food

Body Increases Appetite

Craving to Eat Becomes Irresistible, Resulting in a Binge

Binging Creates Guilt, Purging

BULIMIA

Figure 7-4. *Vicious cycle of a serious eating disorder.*

matized individuals, so the subconscious protected them with a variety of defenses. Wellness returned when the conscious mind accepted reality and dealt with it. The following examples illustrate the process of denial.

Out of Boston comes a horror story about a 15-year-old girl who died of anorexia nervosa. But this was not a simple case of death due to self-starvation. The girl had shown anorexic symptoms at 12. Her surgeon father could not accept anorexia nervosa, a mental illness, as his daughter's diagnosis and so performed exploratory surgery. During her autopsy three years later, 28 exploratory incision scars were revealed. Until nearly the end of his daughter's life the surgeon would not believe that she was emotionally ill.

A 21-year-old bride sat down to the nuptial feast on her wedding day. She consumed everything in sight, then rushed to the restroom. Ten minutes later she emerged from a stall. Her veil, bodice, and sleeves were splashed with vomitus, her satin skirt was dirty from kneeling on the bathroom floor. The groom was in the next room making excuses for his new wife's prolonged absence, just as he had throughout their courtship. Neither he nor she was willing to acknowledge that something was really wrong.

A 16-year-old girl who had weighed 153 pounds at 5 feet 1 inch was brought to a doctor's office weighing 98 pounds. What had looked like healthy weight reduction now frightened her family and friends. But the victim refused to admit she was in trouble. She was sure nothing was wrong and everyone else was overreacting. At 78 pounds, she still insisted that nothing was wrong.

Even among those who have been hospitalized for eating disorders, denial may continue. When a patient alters her true weight by consuming six glasses of water and not urinating before a weigh in or fills her pockets with silverware, it is difficult for the health care team to ascertain whether true gain or loss has occurred.

Codependency and Eating Disorders

The concept of codependency is one of the most exciting and challenging new ideas in the mental health field. Codependency is an illness that develops in people who are lured or trapped into caring for an addicted or self-absorbed person. Codependency is also a way for an insecure person to feel needed in a family or a relationship. A codependent person gives up his or her (usually her) freedom to cater to an addict's insatiable appetite for service and attention, or to pursue the impossible goal of attaining emotional closeness with a distracted or uncaring parent or spouse.

In a codependent person, the virtues of unselfishness and caring are transformed into neurotic drives. The facade of self-sacrifice masks a deep-seated sense of inadequacy.

Because of the inherently unsatisfying nature of the disorder, the codependent person inevitably seeks alternative sources of support. She is most likely to take comfort in behaviors associated with tranquility, like eating. If it helps, the behavior gets repeated. Soon the repetitions become habitual, and then a secondary addiction, or codependency, is created.

Our experience shows that eating disorders caused by codependency occur frequently in families scarred by alcoholism and workaholism. The common factor is inadequate and unreliable emotional support, coupled with high expectations for maturity, independence, and understanding from children and spouses. Both precociously mature children and trapped, drained spouses in these families are victims of chronic emotional deprivation. Neither children nor spouses feel whole, but because they are enthralled by an addict they are unaware of the source of their stress. Instead they blame themselves.

The illness of codependency thrives on ignorance. Codependents are mesmerized by the family's addict: the needy, manipulative person at its core whose own deeply hidden insecurity creates the demand for constant (though often covert) attention.

In middle class families, the development of codependency may be camouflaged by an apparent emotional openness between parents and children, by geographical separation of family members, or even by divorce. The primary addict is often a highly successful male who enjoys wealth and status. He may be at home only rarely, or may be living with his second wife. Nevertheless, his hungry ego is fed by his children's dedication to achievement in school, sports, career, or personal appearance. Even though they may rarely see him, they measure every activity by his standards and generally judge themselves to be short of the mark.

Another source of codependency is the overinvolved parent. This variant we see less often with fathers, but commonly with self-absorbed mothers who do not think of their children as individuals, but as extensions of themselves. In these families the impossible quest for excellence is prompted by the "see how much I do for you" message that is attached to every gift and service rendered. The children learn to devalue their own worth because they believe their well-being depends on parental favors, not responsible caring.

The following example illustrates how codependency operates in a family.

Kerry

Kerry came to the mental health clinic at her college on referral from her mother, who had called before Kerry enrolled to find the "best available help" for her daughter. Kerry had been bulimic for a year, and her parents had known of her symptoms for several months. She had received ineffective outpatient care and antidepressant medication from her local M.D. She had little hope of our being of use to her.

The youngest of three siblings, Kerry told us that her goal in life was to fulfill her father's wish that she make him proud of her. Because her brother and sister were both academically accomplished, Kerry felt she could please him most by being beautiful and feminine.

Kerry had taken her goal to heart in high school, at a time when her father had rarely been home and had been preoccupied with his business affairs whenever he was. Her appearance supported her ambition. She was appropriately thin, wore brightly colored, close-fitted dresses, and maintained a huge, blond coiffure.

Kerry's daily life revolved around the twin goals of maintaining a striking appearance and hanging on academically. Both were difficult goals, and she was chronically anxious and depressed. She used bingeing and purging as a daily source of tension relief. This behavior plus occasional shopping trips to maintain her wardrobe were her sole nonacademic activities.

Although Kerry's behavior seemed superficially self-centered, it took little probing for her to admit that her constant wish was that she make her father happy, and her chronic fear was that she would disappoint him.

Kerry's mother, Estelle, was interviewed to assist in Kerry's treatment. Her own history was a second account of codependency. The daughter of hardworking immigrants, Estelle married Don after their high school graduation. Three children arrived in one, three, and six years. Estelle never developed an identity beyond wife and mother. She learned to contend with Don's preoccupation with business affairs by throwing herself into motherhood.

Although her children were grown, Estelle still catered to their perceived needs and worried about their well-being. But her more basic fear was of being abandoned by her husband. She knew he was unfaithful and came home only to meet his material needs. He was also moody, unpredictable, and demanding. Estelle tried hard not to offend him, and concealed his faults from her family and friends. She saw her role as keeping up appearances, including maintaining a fashionable figure herself. Not surprisingly, Estelle coped with her emotional deficits by eating compulsively and faithfully attending a weight loss clinic. Her lifestyle resembled a low-key, socially acceptable variation of her daughter's.

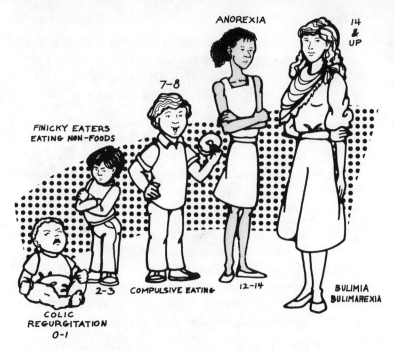

ANOREXIA

14 & UP

7-8

FINICKY EATERS
EATING NON-FOODS

2-3   COMPULSIVE EATING   12-14

BULIMIA
BULIMAREXIA

COLIC
REGURGITATION
0-1

Figure 7-5. *Eating disorders can occur at any age.*

EATING DISORDERS AND AGE

Problems with food take different forms at different ages (Figure 7-5). In the preschool years, an insecure relationship with a primary caretaker, usually the mother, can cause digestive problems in infancy and eating problems later. Colic, regurgitation, and, rarely, projectile vomiting are early signs of trouble. Later, food fads, "finicky" eating, eating nonfood substances, and rumination may occur. (Rumination is bringing up, chewing, and reswallowing previously eaten food.)

The first mature eating disorder is likely to be compulsive eating, which may occur in the early grades. It reflects feelings of isolation and alienation at home or at school. Serious depression at this time typically results in a loss of appetite that may cause severe wasting.

Anorexia is rarely seen before age 11, but often occurs around puberty. Again, the causes are rooted in family conflict at this age, and may represent a struggle for independence, a fear of further maturation, an inexpressible need for affection, or a combination of all three. Children who have been sexually, physically, or emotionally abused are especially prone to developing anorexia at puberty. Also at risk are children with parents who are contemplating separation or divorce.

Families that put a premium on staying fit and keeping thin can induce enough guilt in children from age eight on to cause them to diet compulsively to the degree that physical development is slowed. Such children are not yet eating-disordered, but their fear of failing their parents by becoming fat puts them at great risk for developing such behavior.

Bulimic and bulimarexic symptoms develop in adolescence, with onset peaking twice, around 14 and again about 18. Many therapists have noted that these disorders are triggered by loss or deep disappointment. Laxative and diuretic abuse, the oral expulsion syndrome, and enema abuse seem to occur during older adolescence and adulthood, but there are many exceptions to these norms.

SUMMARY

Problems with food stem from a variety of causes. They are unhealthy and misguided attempts to resolve problems that arise from issues in contemporary culture. Examples of such issues include the following:

Identity Dilemmas

People who are unsure of their full personal worth often focus their attention on their bodies in the hope that achieving an ideal shape or physique will resolve their sense of insecurity. Current fashion places a premium on being extra thin, but trying too hard to lose weight leads to food abuse.

As discussed in Chapter 2, people who believe or have been told that their appearance is especially important for success (actors and models, for example) are particularly at risk. Athletes, dancers, and others who want to fine tune their bodies to reach some ideal or peak of performance, regardless of long-term consequences, are also at risk. These people are often rewarded for maintaining their disorders. For example, ballet dancers are encouraged to be light and lithe. Gymnasts must also maintain a careful food regimen to maintain low weight, and many teachers and coaches willfully overlook how this is achieved. Consequently, young people are introduced to a hazardous activity by persons they view as mentors and role models.

Stress Reduction

Eating is often used to reduce stress. Most young people experience anxiety and depression. It is simply a part of growth and the search for independence and self-identity. Fear of failure or inadequate success, and disappointments with family, friends, and lovers are all too common events. Many anorexic and bulimic episodes are triggered by the loss of a boyfriend or other significant figure and are maintained by chronic loneliness or the fear of being rejected. Stress-induced overeating leads to weight gain, and our cultural obsession with slenderness adds to the initial emotional burden, prompting further abuse of food. Often crash dieting to compensate will set the stage for the onset of binge and purge episodes, or bulimia. Some people feel the act of purging is a catharsis of their stress and anxiety, and find no other activity so immediately gratifying.

Compulsive eating, purging, and fasting have entered the already long list of repetitious behaviors that people adopt as neurotic defenses—like Lady Macbeth's handwashing, or Linus's ritualistic attachment to his blanket. And fat phobia has joined claustrophobia and snakephobia as a disguised expression of more primitive fears that cannot be openly acknowledged.

Sexual Trauma and Fear of Maturity

Many anorexics and bulimics have experienced sexual abuse as children. The trauma causes them to fear sex and hate their own bodies. Often they see self-starvation as as cleansing act. They may come to associate body fat with sexuality and seek to rid themselves of it. They are emotionally unready for adult responsibilities and relationships. By staying underweight, they can postpone accepting an adult identity.

Addictive Behaviors

Food abuse is a type of substance abuse. Starvation (that is, anorexia), binge and purge cycles, and overeating can cause physical and emotional reactions identical to the effects of drugs and alcohol. Young people who grow up in families with drug or alcohol abusing parents or siblings are especially at risk. There are both genetic and environmental reasons for them to drift into food abuse. Eating disorders can become just as entrenched and difficult to resolve as other addictions. The widespread discovery that food can be abused this way is a sad byproduct of the cult of slenderness and a problem that is likely to be around long after being thin becomes passé.

Retreat into Eating Abuse

Adolescents who come from families where being independent and adult is rewarded and where childlike, dependent behavior is discouraged sometimes turn to the comforts eating provides to compensate for feeling alone. Many outwardly successful young people are wracked with hidden anxiety, fearful that they cannot be as strong and resourceful as they believe their parents want them to be. Although they are ashamed of their retreat to infantile eating binges, they find the binges intensely comforting, so they keep them a closely held secret that may go undetected for years. Their parents, deceived into thinking their children are so grown up they do not need much care or attention, pursue other interests. Or they may selfishly create blind spots in their awareness and overlook behaviors that point toward eating disorders because they feel unable to do anything helpful. Being ignored adds to the victim's feelings of isolation and conflict, creating a vicious cycle that increases the isolation and leads to more frequent episodes of food abuse.

A variety of psychiatric disorders are manifested by acting out culturally unacceptable behaviors. The media coverage and notoriety that eating disorders currently receive has made them attention getting, and some people with emotional problems develop eating disorders. They have become "fashionable" symptoms, just as fainting was in the 19th century.

Attention Getting Behaviors

CHAPTER REVIEW

◆ ─────── VOCABULARY ─────── ◆

catharsis the emotional re-enactment in thought or symbolic form of a painful experience that brings relief of the distress the original experience caused.

clinical relating to the practical experience of therapists working with clients.

colic digestive disturbance in newborns and infants.

defense mechanisms thought patterns and behaviors that guard us from painful thoughts and conflicts, thus protecting our sense of well-being.

denial a common and simple defense mechanism whereby destructive behaviors are perceived as harmless; an essential element in all addictive behaviors.

projectile vomiting vigorous involuntary vomiting.

psychoanalysis a school of psychology that interprets human behavior as responses to unconscious motives that reflect early childhood experiences. It was founded by Sigmund Freud and has dominated psychological thought for most of the 20th century.

regurgitation involuntary return of digesting food.

rumination the apparently voluntary regurgitation, chewing, and reswallowing of food.

◆ ─────────FOR YOUR CONSIDERATION─────────◆

◆ The American Psychiatric Association specifies the following
  attributes for a healthy sense of identity:
      Practical long term goals
      Appropriate career choice
      Rewarding friendship patterns
      Secure sense of sexual mores and behavior
      Religious identification
      Moral value system
      Group loyalties.
  A healthy body image is not on the list; but most of us think
  of our appearance as a factor in our identity. Is this an
  important omission? Discuss whether or not body image is a
  vital aspect of a healthy sense of identity.

◆ The body's natural response to starvation is to promote
  appetite. People who are determined to deprive themselves get
  into a battle with their own bodies. Discuss the differences
  between self-discipline and self abuse. Can you develop some
  guidelines that distinguish between these two behaviors?

MARKETING THIN

This chapter will help you:

1. Understand the weight loss techniques marketed by health professionals and commercial operations.
2. Learn that serious limitations apply to all of these programs and that some are truly dangerous.
3. See that healthy weight change can be accomplished, but not with short-term programs or drugs.

♦

"The diet clinic helped me lose weight. Now I'm neurotic about fat and scared to death of food."

The fight to be thin, a battle waged by millions of people, has spawned a multitude of professional and commercial services that offer a wide range of products and advice to people who feel besieged by fat. The slogan "You can never be too rich or too thin" takes on a different meaning when we review the world of weight control. You need to be rich indeed to afford some of the services aimed at making you too thin!

Until quite recently, the quest for a fashionable figure seemed to be a reasonable goal if reasonably pursued. That quest has created a huge marketplace in which all kinds of interested parties compete to sell services. They range from dedicated scientists, concerned health and mental health professionals, and ethical drug suppliers and food manufacturers, to out-and-out quacks who trade on the naiveté and despair of their customers. In the long run, few of these supporting services, whether honorable or not, offer true value for the money. It is quite possible that a person would be better off spending $15 for a mail order plastic running suit to sweat in than spending $1,500 for inpatient treatment at a prestigious teaching hospital. It all depends on what the buyer does with the merchandise.

By and large, weight loss is a self-limiting activity. Even though overweight people are virtually unanimous in claiming they would be happier if they were lighter, the effort required to reduce and stay reduced increases with time, while the added benefits of being thinner decrease as more weight is lost. For most dieters, motivation is hard to sustain.

What usually happens long before the ideal weight is achieved is that the value of losing another pound is perceived as less than the cost in necessary deprivation. At this point, the future looks bleak and punitive, no more weight will be lost, and very soon refeeding will begin, with a return to the original weight, or an even heavier weight, as the end result. The dieter is worse off than before.

Figure 8-1 on the following pages illustrates this phenomenon. It shows that the motivation to lose weight falls as the effort required increases. When the two forces come into balance, the person loses no more weight.

Weight reduction schemes offer a relatively small group of options. But they are marketed in an endless variety of packages, constantly recreating the impression that something new and different has become available. The basic approaches to weight loss include prescription drugs and over-the-counter drugs; intestinal, cosmetic, or oral surgery; diets; behavior modification; psychotherapy; exercise programs; group support; and things that can only be described as outright gimmicks.

Figure 8-1. *Motivation level and the effort required determine when weight loss ends.*

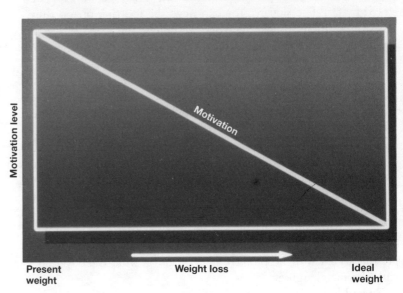

Motivation declines as weight loss continues; it gets harder to stay on the diet; there is less reward for each additional pound lost.

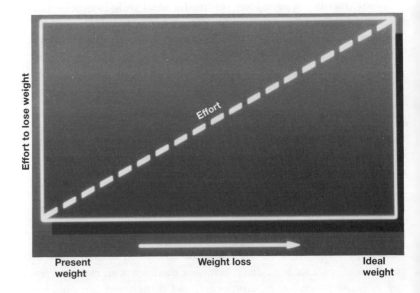

More effort is required for each additional pound lost.

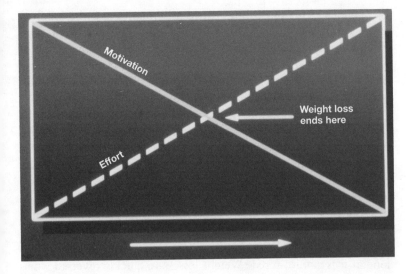

Weight loss ends 〈
the motivation and
effort lines cross.

DRUGS

The pharmaceutical treatment of obesity is by far the most appeal-ing route to thinness because it offers the prospect of effortless weight loss. Also, the association with medicine implies that a cure is being accomplished. Cure implies illness, and most heavy people would rather think of themselves as sick than as undiscip-lined, regardless of whether their condition is the consequence of genes or indulgence.

There is no question that the amphetamines (more accurately called sympathomimetic amines) and related drugs do promote modest, temporary weight loss. There is equally no question that continued use of these drugs fails to produce further losses and that termination of treatment is followed by weight gain.

Maintenance use of these drugs is dangerous. They are marked under a variety of proprietary names: *Dexamyl, Fastin, Pondimin, Preludin, Sanorex,* and *Tenuate* are popular preparations; all are closely related chemically. Although the action of these drugs has been studied extensively, it is still not fully understood. Their use does reduce appetite initially and may increase energy expenditure.

Weight-obsessed patients have long been a stable source of in-come for many physicians in general practice, but they are a gold-mine for doctors in a less respected branch of medicine, bariatrics, who have made weight loss their speciality. These practitioners use

Diet medications that curb appetite are often referred to as anorectics, anorexigenics, or anorexiants.

two major categories of drugs: thyroid hormones and the amphetamines and related drugs. Such practitioners have also tried, with little success, a wide assortment of other preparations, many of which are known to be highly toxic. Perhaps the most notorious of these latter substances is dinitrophenol, which today is most widely used as an insecticide and weedkiller!

The thyroid hormone, which occurs naturally in all healthy people, is available by prescription to increase metabolism and induce weight loss. Unfortunately, most of the weight is lost from muscle tissue, and the hormone causes many other undesirable side effects, some of which can be fatal. Nevertheless, this drug is used as a change agent for a person whose thyroid gland is in good working order, even though continued use may suppress normal secretion of this essential substance.

Extra thyroid unbalances the body's endocrine system only as long as it is administered. Weight losses are quickly reversed when treatment is stopped. And treatment must end if the dangerous side effects are to be avoided. For normal overweight people who have no endocrine disturbance, the drug is useless. The long and fruitless history of this hormone for weight loss in healthy subjects is a striking testimony to the willingness of generations of patients and physicians to substitute wishful thinking for good judgment in the treatment of obesity.

The dangerous side effects of thyroid hormone tend to be long term, but those of amphetamines and related drugs can be more immediate. Because amphetamines induce conditions in the body that mimic a state of alarm or arousal, they may inhibit the digestive functions, causing the body to use fat rather than food for energy.

The most dangerous side effect of amphetamines is increased blood pressure. They also cause heart palpitations, blurred vision, lightheadedness, and dry mouth; long-term use can cause kidney damage and stroke.

The reason their effect is so short-lived may be that appetite reduction is a side effect rather than their principal action. They may work by resetting the body's preferred weight, or setpoint, at a slightly lower level (seldom more than a few pounds). Once the new weight has been achieved, appetite is restored to normal. If this is how they work, and some animal studies support this view, a significant weight loss can only be achieved by increasing the dosage and thus the related side effects. This raises the specter of ever greater dependence on hazardous chemicals.

There is one sympathomimetic amine that is available without a prescription. It is closely related to the prescription amphetamines and apparently is just as effective. It is phenylpropanola-

Hormone and *endocrine* are two words for a class of substances that trigger and control changes in the body's functioning. These substances are produced in glands around the body, and together make up a mechanism called the endocrine system.

mine, or PPA, and is familiar to most consumers as the decongestant in such cold remedies as *Contac, Propagest,* and *Vicks Formula 44D.* It is also approved for sale as an appetite suppressant and is the active ingredient in a host of over-the-counter products like *Dietac* and *Dexatrim.* These products are sold in pharmacies and supermarkets and are misleadingly advertised by mail order companies as a sure cure for fat. Because the Food and Drug Administration (FDA) allows the sale of this substance, advertisers often refer to their product as "Government Approved" or "Federally Tested," implying an endorsement that has never been given.

One especially hazardous weight loss regimen combined amphetamine and thyroid drugs, a procedure previously favored by some physicians. This approach was promoted by drug companies that marketed combination pills for this purpose. The numbers of this type of preparation peaked in the 1960s, when many poorly researched mixtures were marketed. These included the infamous "speedball" combination of amphetamine and barbiturate, which had such a marked effect on the emotions it became a favorite of drug abusers.

Alison

Alison came to our clinic when she was 32, 12 years after she was given her first prescription for amphetamine. An enthusiastic dance student in high school and college, she became terrified of gaining weight as an adult when she saw professional opportunities going to her thinner classmates. The diet pills prescribed by the sports physician at her school worked wonders. She lost her appetite, gained a burst of energy when she took them, and was able to skip dinner to practice. But she soon exhausted the doctor's willingness to prescribe for her. She had lost 20 pounds and her period. She had become dependent on the drugs for the energy she needed to practice and became anxious and sometimes paranoid when their effects wore off. She began to buy drugs from dealers on campus.

Two years later, after a career in dance failed to materialize, Alison trained as a nurse to have access to drugs. For 10 years she lived a roller coaster life, wheedling, lying, stealing, and occasionally dealing to maintain a supply of drugs. Caught several times and fired twice, her life at the periphery of the medical profession was driven by her fear of fat and was dedicated to the quest for amphetamines to kill her craving for food, and sedatives and tranquilizers to quell her chronic anxiety.

Another type of product that was on the market until recently contained a diuretic and a laxative to cause water loss and thus immediate weight change. Health professionals surely were aware that this combination was hazardous and that the results would be instantly reversed when the product was discontinued. Most of these highly toxic combination products have now been outlawed in the United States, but their use continues in countries that have less vigilant regulatory agencies. Wealthy customers who are ready to put their lives on the line for cosmetic gains can find clinics in Mexico that will cater to their fat phobia with heavy doses of these dangerous drugs.

There are two other categories of drugs that have been used as appetite suppressants: bulking agents and topical analgesics. Bulking agents—*Fibre-Trim* (which is advertised for this purpose), *Metamucil*, and *Fiberall* are popular ones—are taken before meals and swell up in the stomach, theoretically creating a sense of fullness that will inhibit excess eating. Benzocaine, a topical analgesic, numbs sensation in the mouth and so makes eating a less rewarding activity. As a weight reducing device you can find it in Slim Line candy and gum. It is our experience that none of these substances provides a lasting change in eating patterns or weight.

Some other over-the-counter medications are used for weight loss, but they are not marketed for that purpose. The most frequently abused are laxatives and diuretics: enemas and emetics are also used. Unfortunately, these substances often work where others fail, but at great risk to health. Laxatives, diuretics, and enemas cause immediate weight loss by reducing the amount of water in the body and food in the digestive tract. They cause further loss by interfering with normal digestion and creating a state of deprivation. By shifting attention from ingestion to defecation, they may inhibit bingeing. They pose both acute and chronic danger because fast evacuation lowers levels of essential chemicals, especially potassium.

Loss of potassium can result in lethal damage to the nervous system, causing heart failure. Weakness, muscle cramps, dizziness, tremors, and irregular heartbeat are common. An individual can move very quickly from minor discomfort to a fatal accident through purgative abuse. Although deaths are not often reported, they can occur without warning. It is likely that some deaths attributed to acute heart disease are precipitated by laxative abuse.

The use of the emetic ipecac to induce vomiting is essentially the same process as purgative abuse. It creates the same hazards, only more acutely. Ipecac is not metabolized as laxatives are. With repeated use, it builds up in the body and can result in serious and fatal nerve damage.

For decades, ipecac syrup has been a staple in first aid kits to induce vomiting after accidental poisoning. Though effective, its use causes acute stomach pain, along with nausea and general misery. It is testimony to the level of fat phobia in our society that women would suffer these noxious effects as an aid to weight loss. In 1985 the FDA and other regulatory agencies held hearings aimed at reducing ipecac abuse by making it a prescription drug. However, it has remained an over-the-counter medication in most states.

Most of these substances lose their effectiveness with constant use. Increasing doses are required to maintain the effects. The side effects become more hazardous as the amount used increases.

RECENT OBESITY "CURES"

Over the years a steady stream of obesity "cures" have found a short-lived moment in the spotlight. Two recent favorites, HCG and starch blockers are substances of varying toxicity that seemed at first to offer a lot based on limited research. They have, however, proved to be ineffective in the long run.

The Hormone HCG

HCG, a hormone extracted from the urine of pregnant women, was typically administered in a daily series of shots accompanied by exhortations and encouragement to stay on a starvation diet. The rationale for this treatment was that weight change during pregnancy is apt to be long lasting. Therefore, by mimicking pregnancy and inducing weight loss, a permanent weight loss might be accomplished. Unfortunately, followup studies demonstrated that HCG patients stayed thin no longer than their peers in other programs.

Protein from Beans

Starch blockers make a virtue out of the familiar problems associated with eating beans. In certain beans, the protein that inhibits starch digestion is concentrated. When this product is taken, it is supposed to inhibit starch digestion and prevent complete metabolism of carbohydrate. It results in malnutrition and possible weight loss at the cost of flatulence and gastric upset. Starch blockers have been taken off the market pending FDA approval.

Steroid Medications

Drugs chemically related to the male hormone testosterone have been used by women to reduce fat deposits. They do this by masculinizing the female body—increasing the proportion of muscle tissue, deepening the voice, coarsening the skin, and promoting facial hair growth. The long-term effects of steroid abuse include severe psychiatric disturbances, osteoporosis, and digestive disorders. Experimenters have found that the relative decrease in fat tissue reverses when the drug is discontinued, but other masculinizing effects tend to be permanent.

The search continues for drugs that will reduce adiposity by controlling appetite or adjusting the setpoint safely and effectively. It is possible that such substances may be developed to relieve the discomfort and handicaps of obesity. It is likely that such drugs will also be used by people who are in good health but feel unattractively heavy.

SURGERY

Four types of surgical intervention are performed for the purpose of weight loss: cosmetic, gastric, intestinal, and oral. We will look at the advantages and disadvantages of each.

Cosmetic Plastic Surgery

Plastic surgery goes directly to the heart of the matter. Unwanted adipose tissue is simply **cut or suctioned** out of the body. Unfortunately, the procedure is more complicated than it might seem.

Fat deposits are not isolated appendages. They are integral parts of the living organism that are joined by connective tissue and embedded in and around muscles, nerves, veins,and arteries. At considerable expense and with some risk, it is possible to reduce the size of these deposits in the arms, thighs, and abdomen with skillful surgery.

Plastic surgery to repair disfigurement and to improve physical proportions has brought relief and renewed self-esteem to many people, but it is not yet possible to remodel a body so that the mundane becomes marvelous. The disadvantages of surgery are:

1. Only a few pounds can be removed.
2. Recovery is painful.
3. Unanticipated side effects are common.
4. Gains may be only temporary.
5. Fat slowly accumulates to replace the lost tissue.
6. Scars from the incisions are permanent.

Altering the Digestive System

A poignant moment on television occurred when Phil Donahue was interviewing fat people. A woman called the show to say her sister had had her stomach stapled and died shortly after the operation. Her voice on the air cut through all our cruel prejudices and shallow vanities about weight when she said, "I only want to say I wish she was still alive."

Gastric and intestinal interventions are limited to very obese patients (Figure 8-2). The many painful and sometimes fatal side effects cannot possibly be justified for people who are not severely handicapped by their adiposity. Such procedures attempt to reduce digestive capacity by shortening the small intestine or by shrinking the effective size of the stomach. Either of these alterations should create a state of semi-starvation and result in weight loss, thought to be a desirable goal for persons who appear to have a chronic positive energy balance and perpetual weight gain. The results of gastric and intestinal surgery have included:

1. A few truly grateful, newly thin persons.
2. Some disappointed people who expected a lot and received a little.
3. Many mutilated people who have had to have surgery reversed to regain their health.
4. Far more fatalities than can be justified for a cosmetic procedure.

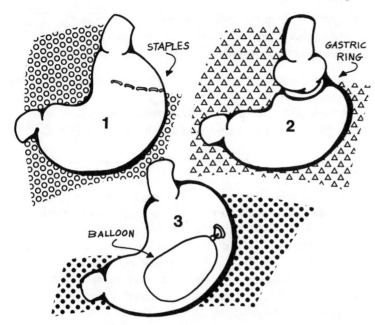

Figure 8-2. Staples, the gastric ring, and the gastric bubble are all used to achieve gastric interruption: 1. Gastric surgery reduces the effective size of the stomach by creating a very small pouch at the entrance. 2. The gastric ring does the same thing with a constrictive band. 3. The gastric bubble achieves the effect by inflating a balloon in the stomach.

Many people who have weight loss surgery suffer from chronic pain, diarrhea, and flatulence. Because their digestive system has been maimed, these people live in a state of constant nutritional deprivation. This state can cause a variety of physical and psychological disturbances that often can only be relieved by reversing the surgery.

Bud

A nurse in Seattle wrote this case history: "When Bud decided to have gastroplasty surgery, he thought his health would improve. Instead, he became critically ill and spent the next year being transferred from one hospital unit to another. . . . During Bud's 10 months with us he went to surgery six times and had almost every conceivable medical and surgical complication. When Bud arrived in the intensive care unit, he *was fitted with an artificial wind pipe, on a ventilator, and heavily sedated. He had a skin ulcer and three gaping, foul smelling abdominal wounds.*

Before stomach stapling, Bud had been a relatively healthy father of four, a 32-year-old factory worker who weighed 450 pounds. His nurse discovered that "he hadn't even wanted to have gastroplasty—he'd been pressured into it by his family and friends."

Over time, the digestive tract may adjust to the surgery and work as effectively as it did prior to the intervention. With physical recovery, however, comes inexorable weight gain.

Two new devices for gastric interruption have been introduced recently. The gastric ring and the gastric bubble were devised to overcome the problems associated with incisions and staples in the digestive tract. The ring, which is clamped around the stomach (see Figure 8-2, p. 139), divides the pouch into two compartments. Food quickly fills the first pouch, creating a sense of fullness before excess intake can occur. The procedure works, but the same side effects that occur with stapling have been observed. Involuntary vomiting, diarrhea, malnutrition, and the various complications of malnutrition still plague patients.

The gastric bubble is similar to the ring but has the advantage of being implanted without surgery. A deflated rubber balloon is inserted through the esophagus and inflated in the stomach. Its presence creates a sense of fullness that may inhibit appetite and eating. Like all prior techniques, the bubble also has limitations. Bursting and deflations create acute hazards requiring emergency removal. Interference in the stomach's normal functions have caused physical damage and illness.

Recommended treatment time for this technique has been shortened to reduce the chance of mishap (which means less weight will be lost). Pounds lost with the bubble will likely be quickly regained when the bubble is removed.

ORAL INTERVENTION

Similar comments apply to another physical intervention: jaw wiring. In this dental procedure, the patient's jaws are loosely connected with stainless steel wires so biting or chewing becomes difficult or impossible, although talking, drinking, and vomiting are less seriously impaired. The necessarily semi-liquid diet is likely to have fewer calories than the patient's regular intake, so some weight is lost. Some people have endured the suffering (not to mention the humiliation) of an imprisoned mouth to enjoy the temporary satisfaction of a thinner figure. Long-term followup studies of this approach are lacking, but there is no reason to suggest the result would be superior to other methods.

Dr. Paul Ernsberger, a neurobiologist and scientific adviser to the National Association to Aid Fat Americans, writes: "**Any** surgical restriction of the flow of nutrients through the stomach will give rise to a set of complications including (but not limited to) anemia, pernicious anemia, osteoporosis, stomach cancer, and premature death. These problems appear in many patients after any of several operations for stomach ulcers, and also appear after stomach operations for weight loss. It is reasonable to conclude that even if 'improved' methods of stomach surgery for weight loss are introduced in the future, they will be likely to cause similar complications, possibly others not foreseen by the surgeon." In a review of the medical literature on weight loss surgery, he concluded that more Americans than were killed in Vietnam (about 53,000) have died as a consequence of these operations.

DIETS

Because there is such a deep conviction in our culture that fatness is linked to overeating, most people believe that changing consumption is the most honest and righteous way to lose weight. It is a short step from there to the conclusion that, if people cannot control their intake alone, they need help from people who are better informed about what it is wise to eat.

Although there is merit in this assumption, there is also a fatal flaw. It lies in the failure to distinguish between guidance and control. We can all profit from education and advice, but we are much less able to profit from the regulation of behavior as intimate and personal as eating.

Many people who believe that their appetites are unhealthy seek to surrender their free will to an authority who will deliver them from themselves. But very few of us are so lacking in self-assertion that we will follow an outsider's rules for long periods. So people rarely follow diets for more than a short time. And the more rigid the requirements of a diet are, the shorter the time people follow them.

A small number of dieters put themselves under the care of the medical profession and spend weeks, sometimes months, in hospitals or health resorts as patients. Often their diet is designed to minimize the loss of muscle and other nonfat tissue, and for that reason is referred to as a **protein sparing modified fast** or **PSMF**.

There is some evidence that PSMF can, at least for awhile, fool the body into shedding more fat than muscle, especially when the diet is supplemented with a rigorous exercise schedule designed to maintain musculature. Such diets are hazardous if they are attempted without close medical supervision. PSMF regimens are currently under intensive study. Carefully balanced, high quality protein diets may ultimately have important clinical applications. But again, as soon as the dieting stops, the weight is regained.

Dietary Aids

Two popular commercial dietary aids should be mentioned: food substitutes sold to increase nonnutritive bulk and liquid formulas designed to be complete replacements for normal meals. In the first category, research has shown that people quickly adjust to disguised changes in the caloric density, richness, or amount of experimental foods, so the body is not long fooled by these substances. The psychological effect of eating tasty low-calorie meals may be a little longer lasting, however, and may help people maintain a regimen of semi-starvation. These meals will not, of course, create a sense of well-being in an underweight person.

The fluid replacement diets that resurface every few years share the same fate as all other rigid modifications in eating behaviors. People generally abandon them after a few weeks when they have lost a few pounds. They then gradually return to their old established patterns.

Nonfood substances that mimic the taste and cooking qualities of sugar and fat are in a developmental stage. One such substance, Simplesse, was marketed in 1988. If any prove to be delicious, inexpensive, and medically safe, they are likely to be viewed as a boon to food lovers and find extensive use. Although it is difficult to predict their effect, we may discover that candy and desserts with low caloric density permit some heavy eaters to indulge without unhealthy weight gain—perhaps getting a satisfaction similar to chewing gum.

One food substitute goes by the unappetizing name of sucrose polyester. Its molecular formula is the mirror image of sugar. It has all the familiar characteristics of sugar, but the human digestive system does not recognize it as food so it passes unabsorbed through the stomach and intestine.

Some research with somewhat less palatable diets showed that people adjust their intake to meet their physiological need for nutrition when the caloric value of their food is decreased. Further, it made no difference how the subjects felt about their shape or weight. This finding suggests that the new nonfoods may merely cause some people to eat more to compensate for their lower energy intake. In doing so, they will revise upward what they assume is a fair amount of eating activity. It should come as no surprise if these developments of the food and drug industry prove to be yet another burden to heavy people, promising much but delivering little.

Regardless of what may show up in the future on the shelves of pharmacies and supermarkets, diets will always have an enduring place among reducing techniques. The reason is that virtually all diets work—for awhile.

There are two principal reasons why short-term weight loss can almost be guaranteed: all diets lower caloric intake so that some starvation occurs, and most of them impose a nutritional shock to the system that the body takes a couple of weeks to adjust to. Thus, both low-carbohydrate and high-carbohydrate regimens will cause brief weight loss. If a diet is in any way diuretic—and most are—the loss of water will increase the apparent weight loss.

So we have the familiar experience of a brief success followed by disheartening failure. Because most people will attribute the success to the diet and the failure to themselves, the net effect is to further reduce the dieter's already low self-esteem, while leaving the diet and its author's reputation unblemished.

Year after year, the weight loss gurus recycle their familiar themes, and the women's magazines publish varieties of quick weight loss programs in issue after issue. Yet nobody points out that if even a fraction of these techniques really worked there would be no need for more new diets.

It is clear that diets as alternatives to free will do not work, but some guidance is needed if we are to make healthy food choices. Dietitians are the helping professionals who are trained for this purpose. In our society, a major part of the economy involves the sale of manufactured food of low nutritional quality. Only the dietitians, working through the media, the schools, and the medical profession, keep us aware of the importance of the four food groups, the hazards of high fat consumption, and the dangers of overprocessed foodstuffs.

Their collective voices serve as a quiet but insistent counterforce to the barrage of expensive advertising that urges us endlessly to buy, to splurge, to indulge, to enjoy, and to risk our health for the benefit of the food industry.

Why Diets Work—For Awhile

The Value of Diets

In raising questions about the value of diets as methods for permanent weight change, we should distinguish between diets that cause caloric deficiency and diets that end caloric overload.

The former are fraudulent in proposing that a single diet, no matter how carefully prepared, can provide for the well-being of persons of varying age, size, health, and metabolic state. The warning, "Check with your doctor before you begin this program" is an escape clause that protects the authors from legal responsibility. (It is not intended to foster an informed debate between patient and physician about the merits of the diet.)

Ending overindulgence, on the other hand, is a much more difficult proposition. Although there can be no doubt that many people abuse food, as others abuse drugs or alcohol, it does not follow that everyone with a big appetite or massive fat deposits is sick or abnormal. If a person's weight has not changed significantly in several years, and if blood pressure and blood sugar are within healthy limits, chances are that the individual is defending (meaning seeking to maintain) his or her proper adult weight.

As discussed in Chapter 3, being substantially overweight does not necessarily decrease life expectancy, and big people are not necessarily overeaters. Some people who crave food and eat a lot may be underweight individuals whose bodies are working to restore lost tissue, even though they are heavier than they would consciously wish to be. Or they could be compensating for a clinical depression, having found that carbohydrates temporarily relieve the emotional lethargy that affects them.

Although many individual differences are normal and are to be respected, not modified, we must consider the plight of people who have overeaten and become obese despite the genetic and regulatory mechanisms of their bodies. Our clinical practice has included many clients who spent years substituting available food for absent affection. Latchkey children are one example. These children habitually fill the lonely hours after school with junk food, candy, and television. Others who experience family tragedies—death, illness, and ugly divorces, for example—often use the pantry as a surrogate parent.

There are many people who are so nutritionally illiterate that they allow their choice of foods to be guided by advertising, convenience, and flavor, virtually without regard to content.

Such people grow fat and stay fat. They have a high risk for hypertension and diabetes, and current medical wisdom concludes that they would be better off thinner. Certainly they would be better off eating nutritionally balanced meals. Careful guidance, both dietary and emotional, is indicated here. Effective treatment must be long-term and individualized. No possible good can come of simple recommendations to go on a diet and lose some weight.

EXERCISE

Increased energy expenditure as the route to weight loss has gained an extraordinary number of enthusiasts in the past decade. There is much evidence that this is a key factor in promoting health and preventing weight gain for many people. Physical fitness through physical activity, which is representative of our cultural ideals, is widely endorsed and is a logical corrective action for self-indulgent behavior.

How better to atone for years of indulgence than by hours of exertion! It may seem foolish, even anti-American to suggest that there are caveats to this concept, but we have come to recognize that the exercise fad is, in part, just another stick to beat the obese with. The fact is that not everyone can, will, or should find salvation in a sweatsuit.

First, however, let us review the benefits. The human frame is roughly divided equally by weight between limbs and the torso. In the 20th century, however, we have witnessed a steadily diminishing need for strong limbs. Enough muscle to get us from our cars to our kitchens and a reserve to take us upstairs to our beds could suffice for our needs. Technology has rendered our limbs almost redundant faster than biology has been able to compensate.

Our response has been to shift from a nation of workers to a nation of exercisers. Through sports and active recreation, we can remain healthy in an environment that tolerates sloth.

Exercise also helps reverse the effects of poor diet. Obese people with slow metabolisms and overeaters with disordered appetites can all experience an easier relationship to food if they exercise. Aerobic exercise (and it is important to stress the need that exercise be aerobic; that is, fat-fueled) increases the basal metabolic rate, reduces appetite, firms muscles, improves cardiac and respiratory function, burns flab, and keeps us out of the kitchen.

Just a few weeks of daily workouts of 30 minutes or so brings these abundant benefits. The resulting sense of well-being is often quite intoxicating. Enthusiastic beginners resolve that they will never be fat or sluggish again; they feel that life has new meaning and value and that their pursuit of happiness has at last been successful.

Organized Programs

Exercise programs vary in quality and appropriateness, and caution is needed in selecting among them. We have had first-hand experience with commercial gyms operated by unqualified personnel, many of whom are fat phobic, compulsive exercisers. To sell memberships, they foster a poor self-image in prospective customers. In their zeal for results, they may urge their clients on in frantic activity to the point of collapse.

Well-run programs employ well-trained people, preferably people whose income does not depend directly on the number of people they recruit. The focus is on health first and appearance second, and careful individual assessment precedes any strenuous activity. Very few commercial gyms meet these criteria. Nonprofit organizations like the YMCA and YWCA and employer-sponsored fitness programs are more likely to have the right priorities, but even here staff members may be underqualified or overenthusiastic.

Why Some People Exercise and Some People Don't

It is true that the mass discovery of the benefits of physical fitness has virtually guaranteed that our public health statistics are going to improve in the coming years, but not everyone is able to enjoy these benefits. Many people who experience all the positive rewards of exercise still fall back to a familiar sedentary routine and regain the weight they have lost.

We believe that there are two major reasons for this, the first is based on population statistics and the second is based on variations in body type.

North Americans and Europeans have been influenced by the enormous rise in the birth rate that followed World War II. As this bulge of humanity has moved from the cradle to the grave, it has continued to dominate our economic and social environment. What happened in the 1970s and is continuing to influence the 1980s is that babies born in the 1940s and 1950s have aged to the point where bountiful health is no longer an unearned benefit. As they pass their mid-20s the strength, speed, and svelte that graced their youth diminish. Their response is typical of the work ethic that is still the keystone of our culture: They begin an endless struggle to hold back the march of time.

Today, we are still at that point where most people believe that earnest exercise is the price of well-being. And for many it indeed is. Others of us, however, have accepted social and professional responsibilities that quite simply diminish the possibility for vigorous exercise. Torn between the multiple demands on us, we relegate active recreation to a minor role. Regardless of the benefits it promises, there is a limit to how far we are willing to follow fashion.

The second major reason why not everyone will exercise is that only persons with certain kinds of physique find voluntary activity invigorating (Figure 8-3). As described in Chapter 6, the human body can be categorized according to three criteria: soft and rounded (endomorphic), square and muscular (mesomorphic), and thin and bony (ectomorphic).

The degree to which people take naturally to exercise depends on how muscularly endowed, or mesomorphic, they are. Predominantly endomorphic and ectomorphic people are reluctant athletes, poor performers, and early quitters. The mesomorphs, on the other hand, cannot be kept home for long—their need to be active is constant, pressing, and dominant. As far as they are concerned, the more activity the better.

The search for slimness rarely takes these variables into account. Although the inactive ectomorph is rarely condemned, the unmuscled endomorph who finds no pleasure or success in competition is continually urged to get out there and exercise.

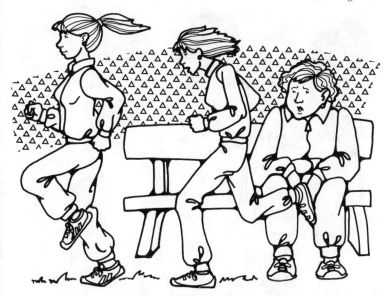

Figure 8-3. Exercise doesn't have the same effects on persons with different body types. What kind of exerciser are you?

Of course, relatively few people have extreme forms of body type. Most of us are midrangers with a blend of all three characteristics. Even so, however, our temperament is likely to reflect our predominant body type. The amount of satisfaction we take in activity is related to our degree of mesomorphy.

Sometimes the programs inflicted on the obese border on punishment. An "experiment" at the University of Pennsylvania seemed especially so. Heavy women subjects were required to pedal exercise machines while submerged to their necks in cold water. This humiliating activity was continued for an hour a day, five days a week for six weeks. No weight loss was recorded, probably because the womens' bodies avoided hypothermia by maintaining their fat stores.

GROUP TREATMENT

This is a good place to note how cruelly our present culture treats endomorphy. Fat people suffer in three ways: because the high levels of refined carbohydrate, sugar, and fat in the typical American diet make them heavier, because mechanization has limited their opportunities for enforced daily energy expenditure, and because fashion has identified them as homely. It takes courage to be overweight in America today, a courage that millions have sought by joining groups formed to aid in weight loss.

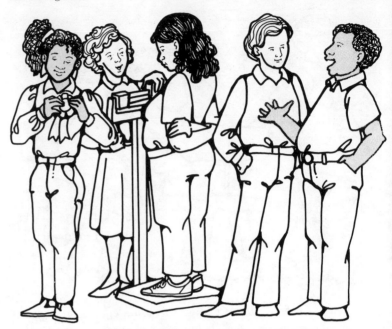

Figure 8-4. *Self-help groups are a popular approach to short-term weight loss; long-term reduction is less certain.*

Group treatment for weight reduction ranges from informal get togethers among friends and neighbors to multimillion dollar organizations like Weight Watchers. These groups are formed by heavy people seeking support in the battle with their bulges, by researchers collecting information, by health professionals offering help, by profit-oriented corporations marketing programs and promises, and by various combinations of these people.

Some of the self-help groups have become international organizations: Take Off Pounds Sensibly (TOPS) and Overeaters Anonymous (OA) have grown steadily for over 20 years and have been havens of help for many. Weight Watchers, the giant of the commercial operations, now operates worldwide. Other programs are run by medical centers, colleges, YMCAs, and individual entrepreneurs (Figure 8-4).

Most of these operations have two things in common: they bring overweight people together and they promote standard procedures to combat fat. One exception is OA, which is concerned with overeating not overweight, although weight loss is not discouraged.

Our concern with these programs is that they are too ready to offer service to anyone who wants to join. The clientele is self-selected, and the assumption tends to be that if a person **feels** overweight then he or she **is** overweight, and treatment will be initiated. It follows that the goals that are established are guided more often by cosmetics than by physiology, and the hazards of excess weight loss are virtually ignored.

One consequence of the procedures is that the programs may induce eating disorders in people who, prior to treatment, had no illness or disease, and were not clinically obese or unhealthy. The net effect of such weight loss is likely to be an aroused appetite, unwanted weight gain, panic, and a second round of treatment.

Irresponsible weight reduction procedures from which this sequence of events follows have a built-in bonus for the commercial operators. Customers frequently seek to be recycled through the program, unaware that the prior treatment they received contributed to their present misery. No weight loss program ever admits this. Most, in fact, stress the permanence of their results. But there is little if any evidence to back up their claims. They always welcome back old clients who want to start over.

We do not know how much these big operations depend on repeat business. But, to the extent that the programs create future clients by training people to unbalance their metabolisms, they are profiting by making people sick.

By and large, the group programs offer some mix of diet, exercise, and behavior modification presented in a social context that blends mutual support with competition. Leaders who can inspire just the right mix of these ingredients create a highly motivating atmosphere in which dispirited fat people find acceptance, challenge, and renewed self-esteem.

Powerful, positive experiences, both emotional and physical, are realized, and participants may learn to feel good about themselves for the first time in years. Many success stories begin, "It started when I joined the XYZ weight control program . . ."

Group treatments that maximize these gains and make careful assessments of individual needs may be excellent therapeutic mechanisms. There is a great need for caution in selecting programs, however, because many offer far more than they deliver. Few consumers have the expertise to evaluate programs. To our knowledge, no professional organization or licensing authority exists to certify or license programs.

> Remember, when we use the term "overweight" we are referring to how people perceive themselves, and not to some arbitrarily set number of pounds.

> How many women do you know who lost weight, met their husbands, married at the lightest weight of their adult lives, and then returned to their previous size, to their own and their mate's dismay?

BEHAVIOR MODIFICATION

Behavioral treatments were the high flyers of the 1970s. The idea, in a nutshell, is to train people to abandon unhealthy eating behaviors and adopt healthy ones. The changes are accomplished by introducing a system of rewards, and sometimes punishments, plus alterations in the patient's environment. People are usually weaned away from junk foods and snacks, trained to eat reasonable meals at accepted mealtimes, and taught to develop a repertoire of activities that are substitutes for eating.

Many effective programs were developed using these concepts (we discuss one, called STEM, in Chapter 10) and for awhile it seemed that the key to controlling obesity would be found in the perfection of this approach.

Long-term followups, were rarely done, however, and those that were done proved disappointing. Like all the other interventions, behavior modification was a short-term success and a long-term failure for most people who tried it.

We believe that there are two factors involved with the failure of behavior modification. First, attempting to alter a healthy, if unfashionable, organism mobilizes powerful recuperative responses that will restore the pre-existing equilibrium. The body will demand weight gain. Second, behavioral therapists have access only to the relatively superficial aspects of their patients' lives. When treatment ends, entrenched patterns of behavior reassert themselves.

Behavioral treatments work best when early gains open the way to further improvements in living; for example, when successful sex therapy leads to an enhanced marriage. Losing weight might seem to fit this model, but for many people it does not. The early pleasure associated with being thinner usually gives way to a realization that life has not changed all that much, and staying thin turns out to be a constant struggle. Given this outcome, relapse is almost inevitable.

Only people who truly change their lives for the better succeed in maintaining substantial weight loss, and then only for as long as their newly enhanced status depends on staying thin.

PSYCHOTHERAPY AND HYPNOTHERAPY

Mental health therapists are frequently sought out by "overweight" and obese patients on the assumption that an emotional problem has caused them to be fat. For people who have gained weight as adults, and as a consequence of identifiable stresses, such a referrral is entirely appropriate. It may also be wise to seek a psychological evaluation if only to rule out the possibility that the unwanted fat may have been gained because of emotional problems.

Unfortunately, not many therapists are well informed about these matters, and there is a tendency in the mental health profession to presume that emotional health correlates with a fashionably attractive appearance.

Therapists who can identify realistic physical and dietary goals and can then assist their clients over the emotional hurdles impeding them may be crucial figures in restoring or enhancing their patients' health. In the buyer beware climate that pervades psychotherapy today, finding a therapist who is both adequately trained and personally compatible is apt to be a matter of trial and error.

These cautions need to be reiterated more forcefully when applied to hypnotherapy—a healing art with a justifiable reputation for quackery, as well as a core of qualified and effective practitioners. Treatment to promote weight loss is a stock-in-trade of virtually all hypnotherapists, and short-term changes in eating behaviors are not difficult to achieve by using posthypnotic suggestion. The effect, however, is rarely lasting unless it is accompanied by therapy that brings insight, understanding, and emotional growth. These gains are unlikely to occur unless the therapeutic relationship is based on more than a facility for trance induction. Check very carefully before seeking help of this nature.

> We urge people who are seeking treatment to feel free to check a number of potential therapists, and to ask direct questions about their knowledge of eating and appetite disorders before committing themselves to a course of treatment.

Last, and by all means least, we should mention and quickly dismiss all gadgets, gimmicks, and garments that are sold—almost always by mail order—to "melt" fat in minutes a day without pain or effort. The utterly ineffective varieties on the market include items like inflatable pants, rubber corsets, and plastic overalls. Faintly less fraudulent, but no more likely to be effective, are the exercise wheels, rope and pulley devices, elastic cords, and cheap pedaling machines that are billed as being capable of transforming one's body if used briefly but conscientiously on a regular basis.

GIMMICKS

Exercise does have value in health maintenance, but the mechanisms themselves have no special therapeutic effect. They are usually so cheaply made that they break before any benefit from their use could accrue.

In this context, we should mention two other kinds of mechanical exercisers—one group that works and one that does not. Included in the group that works are the quality built stationary bicycles, rowing machines, and treadmills that are found in any well-equipped gymnasium, and that can be purchased for home use. Such machines are costly but effective, and using them properly—which means with considerable effort—will improve physical fitness and may induce weight loss.

We do not include weight training equipment in this category because it is most often, and most effectively, used for non-aerobic exercise, which has no value for weight reduction.

The expensive machines that do not provide meaningful assistance, but are nevertheless popular, are the passive "exercisers" and massagers. Commercial slimming salons—establishments which themselves are often no more than large-scale gimmicks— use these electric-powered rollers, vibrating belts, and whirlpools. Although they are fun to play with, may give an invigorating massage, and may even have value in physical therapy, they will not promote weight loss.

Similarly ineffective devices are saunas, hot tubs, mud packs, body wrappings, and all the other constantly changing offerings that wax and wane in popularity over the years. Enjoy them by all means, but do not imagine that they have benefit beyond the immediate sense of well-being and relaxation they create.

SUMMARY

In the western world, the desire to be thin has created a huge market for techniques that presume to help people shed fat tissue. New medical, psychological, behavioral, and dietary interventions are introduced almost daily in a bewildering array. Some are developed by scientists with detailed knowledge of the problem, but the vast majority are invented and sold by unqualified people with a flair for promotion and marketing. Virtually all techniques cause minor initial weight loss, followed by regain. Many are hazardous to health. Only interventions that help people make permanent healthy changes in their lifestyles are truly effective.

DANGEROUS WEIGHT LOSS METHODS
THROUGH THE AGES*

1862   Low-carbohydrate diet introduced. Remains one of the most popular reducing regimens today.

1893   Pharmacological doses of thyroid extract first used.

1920's   First fad diets: Hollywood (Melba toast) diet, grapefruit diet.

1920's   Laxatives promoted as weight reducing remedies.

1933   Dinitrophenol introduced.

1935   After reports of severe and sometimes fatal side effects, the AMA withholds its approval of dinitrophenol.

1936   100,000 obese Americans have taken dinitrophenol, which is widely available by mail order. Usage declines gradually over the next decade.

1937   Amphetamine introduced as weight loss treatment, and quickly comes into widespread use.

1940   Digitalis introduced for weight loss in doses high enough to produce nausea. Digitalis remains a common treatment for obesity for 30 years, a use that persists today.

1940   Atropine introduced as a weight loss medication in combination with sedatives.

1946   Multiple-drug weight-loss regimens become popular. Examples include a combination of thyroid, amphetamine, sedatives, and digitalis administered to fat children, and a combination of amphetamine, thyroid, and diuretic. This "rainbow pill" approach remains popular for nearly 25 years, and persists today among some bariatric physicians.

1948   Two-thirds of all patients treated for overweight are given amphetamines.

1953   The low-carbohydrate diet reintroduced as the Pennington or DuPont diet.

1959   The Build and Blood Pressure study is released, triggering an upsurge in prescriptions for diet pills, and stimulates professional and lay interest in weight control.

1959   Total fasting in a hospital setting is introduced.

1961   *Calories Don't Count* again reintroduces the low-carbohydrate diet, sells over 2 million copies, spawns scores of imitators, and establishes the dominance of the low-carbohydrate diet for the next quarter of a century.

1964   Total fasting for prolonged periods (up to 4 months) is put into practice.

(Continued on next page)

1969	Widespread use of intestinal bypass begins.
1971	Juice fast is popularized. Faddists claim that subsistence solely on juice for up to 100 days is safe.
1974	Jaw wiring is put into widespread use.
1976	*The Last Chance Diet* convinces millions to try the protein-sparing modified fast.
1977	The surgical staple gun allows the widespread use of gastric bypass.
1979	Phenylpropanolamine approved by the FDA as an over-the-counter diet pill.
1979	Four million Americans have gone on a liquid protein diet.
1980	An estimated 30,000 gastric bypass operations are performed annually.
1980	Calling the best-selling ultra-low-calorie Cambridge Plan a "serious risk to health", the U.S. government files suit to ban sales. Legal action is blocked when the diet is sold by direct market, rather than through the mails. Within four years, 7 million fat Americans will have used this diet.
1981	*The Beverly Hills Diet* teaches millions of dieters to eat large quantities of fruit in order to cause severe diarrhea and thus weight loss.
1982	Despite widespread condemnation by medical authorities, or perhaps because of its notoriety, *The Beverly Hills Diet* begets a bestselling sequel.
1982	An estimated 50,000 gastric bypass operations are performed annually.
1983	The highly popular Herbalife Slim and Trim Formula is the subject of an action by the FDA. The product contained the highly toxic herbs mandrake and pokeroot in an ultra-low-calorie formula diet. Herbalife annual sales are claimed to be over 55 million dollars.
1985	The FDA approves the gastric balloon as a medical device for inducing weight loss.
1986	Following complaints of severe and even fatal side effects, and questions regarding efficacy, the FDA re-investigates the gastric balloon.

*From "Rethinking Obesity: An Alternative View of Its Health Implications." Paul Ernsberger and Paul Haskew, Human Sciences Press, New York (1987).

CHAPTER REVIEW

◆ ──────── VOCABULARY ──────── ◆

aerobic   fat-fueled; aerobic exercise increases basal metabolic rate, reduces appetite, firms muscles, improves cardiac and respiratory function, and burns flab.

amphetamines   drugs frequently prescribed to promote weight loss. Such loss is temporary, however, and termination of treatment is followed by weight gain.

anorectics   name frequently used for diet medications that curb appetite.

defending   seeking to maintain one's proper adult weight.

gastric bubble   a rubber balloon inflated in the stomach to create a sense of fullness.

gastroplasty   surgical procedure to reduce digestive capacity by shortening the small intestine or shrinking the effective size of the stomach.

purgatives   a substance or method used to eliminate food before it can be digested.

◆ ──────── FOR YOUR CONSIDERATION ──────── ◆

◆ The evidence presented in this chapter testifies to the general failure of weight reduction techniques and programs of all kinds to provide long term loss. Nevertheless, billions of dollars are spent on them, and medical practitioners frequently recommend weight reduction treatments. What personal experiences have you had with weight loss? Do they confirm or contradict what you have read? Discuss whether legislation regulating commercial weight loss enterprises would be in the public interest.

◆ Have you known anyone who tries every diet and gimmick that comes along in the hope of losing weight? How successful is this practice? What, if anything, would help this person? What message does such behavior convey?

CHAPTER

9

THERAPY FOR EATING DISORDERS
The Search for Understanding

This chapter will help you:

1. Trace the history of treatments for anorexia and bulimia.
2. Understand the effect reports in the media can have.
3. Know the benefits and problems associated with inpatient and outpatient care for eating problems.
4. Recognize that, despite progress in treatment, many victims of eating disorders still receive inadequate care.
5. Find how to get the best available care in your locality.

◆

"The first two therapists I went to couldn't believe that eating was my problem. They wanted to talk about everything else in my life except food!"

The appetite disorders that cause a severe underweight state or bizarre eating behaviors have not yet given rise to commercially oriented therapies. These disorders are still alien and a little scary, and their victims lack the visibility and familiarity that characterize the obese. Healthy people have more difficulty relating sympathetically to behavioral and emotional problems than they do to physical disease and illness. Victims rarely talk about their problems, and as most look healthy, the public is largely unaware of the incidence of the disorder.

These facts have served to preserve a cloak of secrecy and a sense of mystery over behaviors that in reality are neither uncommon nor as frightening as, say, chronic drunkenness or reckless driving.

The low level of public and professional understanding of appetite disorders leads to abnormal anxiety. Many therapists, aware that anorexia nervosa is a potentially lethal condition, are reluctant to offer treatment to a person who starves herself. In contrast, they do not hesitate to accept a depressed patient who is actively contemplating suicide.

Again, until recently, bulimia was believed to be a rare and dangerous phenomenon that was unlikely to be encountered in clinical practice. As a consequence, these expectations became self-fulfilling: bulimics believed they were unique and stayed out of treatment programs.

In the past, most pathorexics did not seek treatment, and those who did tended to be in extreme distress. Neither the professionals nor the public realized that behind facades of middle class normality, hundreds of thousands of Americans were existing in various states of semi-starvation or were engaging in massive overeating and purging cycles. And, for the most part, the people involved in these practices thought they were alone, trapped in behavior patterns they could not change, and convinced that no one would accept them if they told the truth about themselves.

A major change in public awareness of eating disorders occurred in 1981, when many newspaper articles and television programs about bulimarexia appeared. *Newsweek,* in its year-end issue, facetiously referred to 1981 as "the year of the binge-purge syndrome." In some adolescent circles, girls who were known to vomit gained status, and the expletive *barf!* became popular and gained a positive as well as negative connotation.

Attitudes toward food and eating have shifted dramatically with the growing awareness of how potentially hazardous eating disorders can be. Bingeing has found a place in the repertoire of teenage activities that cause parents sleepless nights. It is still too soon to determine what effects these changes have had.

THE IGNORANCE SURROUNDING EATING DISORDERS

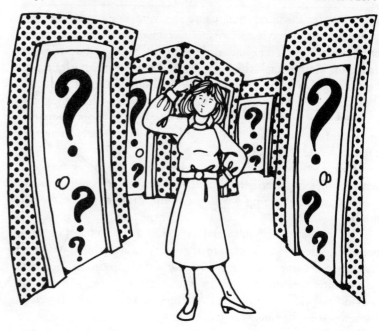

OVEREATERS ANONYMOUS

A long-time exception to the general ignorance about eating disorders has been the growing group of people who find relief in the care and understanding of Overeaters Anonymous (OA), an organization modeled on the teaching and practices of Alcoholics Anonymous. Members of OA acknowledge that when they are alone, they are powerless in the face of their desire to eat compulsively. They recognize that weight is not the issue; eating is the problem.

The parallels between compulsive eating and alcohol abuse are many and close, and the two organizations have helped many thousands of people regain self-respect and a sense of control over their lives. Most OA members are fat, but not all. There is much empathy, understanding, and support for all appetite-disordered people. OA has become a major therapeutic resource for pathorexics of all kinds. You locate meetings by calling OA. Numbers are listed in all major city telephone directories, and in many others also.

It is important to recognize that OA is a nonprofessional self-help group run by and for its members, who are all self-diagnosed compulsive eaters. They do not presume to make medical or technical judgments about each other. This fact represents both the strength and the weakness of OA: strength, because all leadership is based on personal knowledge and experience; weakness, because some OA members perpetuate their disorders by striving to stay

THE TWELVE STEPS

1. We admitted we were powerless over alcohol (food)—that our lives had become unmanageable.

2. Came to believe that a Power greater than ourselves could restore us to sanity.

3. Made a decision to turn our will and our lives over to the care of God *as we understood Him.*

4. Made a searching and fearless moral inventory of ourselves.

5. Admitted to God, to ourselves and to another human being the exact nature of our wrongs.

6. Were entirely ready to have God remove all these defects of character.

7. Humbly asked Him to remove our shortcomings.

8. Made a list of all persons we had harmed, and became willing to make amends to them all.

9. Make direct amends to such people wherever possible, except when to do so would injure them or others.

10. Continued to take personal inventory, and when we were wrong, promptly admitted it.

11. Sought through prayer and meditation to improve our conscious contact with God *as we understood Him,* praying only for knowledge of His will for us and the power to carry that out.

12. Having had a spiritual awakening as the result of these steps, we tried to carry this message to alcoholics (compulsive overeaters) and to practice these principles in all our affairs.

Reprinted with permission of AA World Services, Inc., PO Box 459, Grand Central Station, New York, NY 10017

constitutionally underweight and receive unconditional support from fellow members for their oftentimes misguided efforts.

Members who have been abstinent for awhile may choose to work through a program of twelve steps toward a greater freedom from addiction. The immense success that has been achieved with the twelve steps has prompted many other therapeutic organizations, clinic, and hospitals to adopt or promote them. They then refer to themselves as Twelve Step programs. However, the steps originated with Alcoholics Anonymous, and AA does not license or approve their adaptation for other purposes. They are given in the accompanying box in their original form, with Overeaters Anonymous' variation printed in parenthesis.

Many of our clients have been greatly helped by OA. One who perhaps typifies the best outcome is Cathy, a housewife with two preschool children, who believes that OA saved her marriage and maybe her life.

Cathy

"*I was always careful about my weight, but when I got pregnant with Jimmy, my second son, the doctor said I should gain some more weight to be on the safe side. That really panicked me, and of course I did just the opposite! . . . Then when I was home from the hospital, all I could think about was food. There was nobody around, I felt really lonely, and somehow I started eating crackers and spitting them out. Once when I did that, I gagged and threw up. I was crying when it happened.*"

Within days of that experience, Cathy was eating crackers nonstop and pausing to throw up every 20 minutes. The behavior continued for three years and hardly changed, even after she began psychotherapy.

Cathy became sickly and depressed, and her marriage deteriorated. She rarely left home except to buy food. Finding plausible reasons for buying cartons of crackers became a troubling preoccupation. That, perhaps more than anything else, precipitated her decision to seek therapy.

With our encouragement, Cathy contacted OA. Fortunately, her sponsor (the contact person assigned to a new member) had had her own brush with bulimarexia. She knew how much support Cathy would need in the beginning. She helped Cathy substitute telephone calls for saltines—10 to 15 separate calls a day in the first month. Gradually, Cathy was weaned from her dependency, and her life returned to normal. But OA is still important to her, both for the support she gets and for the help she now gives to others.

PROFESSIONAL ORGANIZATIONS

During the 1970s, three organizations formed to help eating-disordered people: the National Association for Anorexia Nervosa and Associated Disorders, Inc. (ANAD); the American Anorexia/ Bulimia Association (AA/BA); and the National Anorexia Aid Society (NAAS). These groups combine lay energy with professional input. The addresses and telephone numbers of these organizations are listed in Appendix B.

In 1985, a group of therapists organized to share information and establish minimum standards for eating disorder counselors. They became the International Association of Eating Disorders Professionals (IAEDP) and are listed in Appendix B. The Association helps publicize the fact that eating disorders are recognized and treatable phenomena that have been known for decades and have been treated successfully in hospitals, outpatient clinics, and therapists' offices.

These organizations also offer forums for parents and spouses of victims by setting up meetings where affected people can share their experiences. The anguish of watching helplessly or battling fruitlessly while a child or loved one is trapped in an eating disorder no longer needs to be a lonely vigil.

THE HISTORY OF TREATING EATING DISORDERS

Medical treatment of eating disorders has been available since they were diagnosed and named (Dr. William Gull first used the term anorexia nervosa in London in 1874). Until the 1960s, the vast majority of anorexics were hospitalized on medical, not psychiatric, wards. Before the development of antibiotics, wasting disorders were taken much more seriously. Infectious diseases like pneumonia took the lives of many young people who had insufficient fat stores to survive through the course of their illness.

Hospital records show that in the 1930s anorexic patients were **admitted** to hospitals at weights higher than weights they currently are **discharged** at. The treatments were not effective, however. Forced feeding and punitive incarceration featured too prominently as therapy to give anorexics much assurance that they would be cared for with genuine sympathy. Though we can sense the frustration of hospital staffs confronted with patients who seem bent on self-destruction, we know now that coercive techniques are generally counterproductive. They do nothing to promote long-term improvement and growth in self-respect.

In the 19th century and the first half of the 20th century, psychiatry often had to be content to offer diagnosis rather than treatment to the emotionally ill. Supportive care was its principal form of treatment. Psychoanalysis and some rival but closely related philosophies of personality provided penetrating insights into the role of unconscious motives in determining human behavior. Unfortunately, applying these discoveries to patient care proved very expensive, and the results were disappointing.

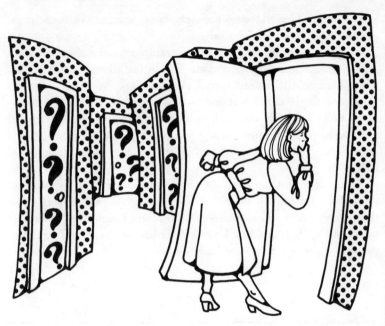

Nevertheless, psychoanalytic therapy dominated the profession. The result was that anorexics (bulimics were still too rare to draw the attention of therapists) received a diagnostic straightjacket that labeled them afraid of adult sexuality. They were simply thought to be delaying maturation through deliberate malnutrition.

To be sure, many sensitive therapists were able, with care and understanding, to help patients recover from their disabling symptoms. Also, we should acknowledge that sexual fears often are present in anorexia. But we now recognize that self-starvation is a symptom that attaches itself to many emotional disorders and also to some physical ones.

People with eating disorders still have a reputation for yielding only to therapists with acute empathy and insight, keeping alive the self-fulfilling expectation that they are somehow special problem people who need extra special attention.

In the 1950s and 1960s, the pioneering work of some now famous therapists and researchers greatly expanded our knowledge of treatments for eating disorders. Hilde Bruch, Salvatore Minuchin, and Maria Selvini-Pallazzoli, to name three, all helped to identify the social context in which eating disorders occur. Their example shifted the treatment focus from the individual to the family. Few therapists today would consider working with an adolescent anorexic without having the parents, and maybe the siblings, in some form of treatment also.

Until the 1970s, bulimia and bulimarexia were generally assumed to be variants of anorexia nervosa. This was therapeutically unfortunate and served to suppress both the treatment options and the identification of patients. Much credit is due Marlene Boskind-White, who, as a psychologist at Cornell University in 1974, described and named bulimarexia.

She developed a successful therapy that addressed her patients' overly compliant femininity and broadened and strengthened their sense of identity. Her concepts revolutionized treatment goals and greatly increased the number of people seeking help.

Meanwhile, the physiology of eating and appetite has become better understood. Until recently, few people questioned the notion that we are free to choose how wide we want to be. It was presumed to be simply a matter of deciding how much fat to carry. Although we now know that this is false, we are not sure just how false it is. Some variables that control appetite and adiposity have been identified and are discussed thoroughly in Chapters 6 and 7.

TREATMENT TODAY

Much more information about physiology and nutrition awaits clarification. Because we know that this knowledge will have a major impact on treatment goals and therapy, we can expect strategies to help pathorexics to evolve quickly in the light of new findings. So fresh is this field that a meeting in New York in 1982 was billed as "the first annual conference . . ." on the treatment of anorexia and bulimia. Another landmark was publication in the fall of 1981 of the first issue of the *International Journal of Eating Disorders.*

Now that there is widespread public awareness of pathorexia, the number of people seeking treatment increases daily. Many therapists have received orientation and training to meet the unprecedented demand for service, and eating disorder clinics have been organized at many psychiatric hospitals and mental health centers.

If you are looking for a clinic or therapist in your neighborhood, you can call any of the organizations listed in Appendix B for names of people known to be well versed in problems with food. Another good source of information may be the mental health service or counseling center at a local college or university. You may get a referral to a respected therapist by asking for suggestions at an Overeaters Anonymous meeting, or by calling local medical doctors. Counselors and clinics listed in the Yellow Pages under "Marriage and Family Counselors" and "Psychologists" often specify their interest in treating eating disorders—but that is no testimony to their competence.

Regardless of your source of referral, or the reputation of your therapist, you are the judge of whether the treatment is helpful. Do not stay in therapy if you sense a lack of understanding, empathy, or knowledge. An effective therapist will address painful issues and may not always leave you feeling at peace with yourself; but your distress will be related to the problems you are working on, not the relationship with your therapist.

Because of the addictive nature of eating disorders, many inpatient facilities run programs that have a lot in common with proven alcohol and drug abuse treatments. There is a heavy emphasis on learning about the nature of eating disorders. Groups of patients work together to build self-esteem and to solve other personal problems. Family sessions help restore support and affection and help undercut destructive competition and other negative traits. All treatment centers offer individual counseling; many use medication to help relieve physical symptoms, to restore a sense of calm, or to normalize moods.

Even though specialized hospitals and clinics have been formed throughout the country, many—perhaps most—anorexic and bulimic inpatients are still treated in general hospitals and psychiatric facilities, where the quality of care varies widely with the expertise of the staff. Some psychiatric wards do very well with their eating-disordered patients, but there are many exceptions. Anorexics can get into power struggles with their psychiatrists and be discharged at a lower weight than they were admitted at because the hospital does not want a patient in its care to starve to death.

Bulimic patients on general psychiatric wards often seem quite mysterious to their fellow patients and to the staff. When it becomes clear that they can maintain their symptoms no matter how closely they are monitored, they are apt to be left alone with their illness and treated with an array of medications in the hope of finding something that will work. After a few months the symptoms do abate and the patient is discharged. In most cases the bulimia resumes shortly afterwards.

The vast majority of eating disorder victims are never hospitalized. The care they receive is in a doctor's or therapist's office, and again varies a great deal in effectiveness.

A constantly recurring tragedy finds young women desperate for help with uncontrollable bulimia getting inadequate or unsympathetic attention from health professionals who fail to grasp how seriously ill their patients are. The disappointing outcome often discourages victims from looking again for more competent care. We hope that as awareness of eating disorders grows and both professionals and the public learn more about the availability of treatment, these personal catastrophes will become rare.

The course of successful treatment for eating disorders ranges from a few sessions to many years of both in- and outpatient care. The time required for recovery depends on many variables, the three most important being the severity of symptoms, the length of time before treatment is initiated, and the kind of relationship established between patient and therapists.

The first two variables are measures of how entrenched the pathology is. Although the third variable, the therapeutic relationship, is harder to gauge, it is just as important. Perhaps more than anything else, problems with food call for empathy, understanding, and patience. Typically, food problems are symptoms of developmental disorders, meaning that the normal process of growth and maturation has gone awry. It takes decades for healthy human development to occur. Repairing serious flaws is similarly slow, even when it is steady. So effective treatment may require several years of work with a therapist who stays in close touch with the patient.

Happily, however, not all eating disorders are deeply rooted. Millions of people experience brief episodes that resolve without professional care. Others gain insights from a few sessions with a well-trained counselor, or even from a well-written book or magazine article, that are sufficient to relieve their problems.

In the long run, prevention of eating disorders is far more important than cures. It is our hope in writing this book that the hazards of food abuse and the no-win nature of punitive dieting will become more widely understood. Armed with that knowledge, and prepared to avoid entrapment in the cult of slenderness, young people can make the specter of eating disorder a matter for history books instead of health texts.

SUMMARY

Therapy for eating and appetite disorders has evolved from medically oriented weight restoration, through care focused on psychoanalysis, to broadly based in- and outpatient services that respond to the varied nature of these illnesses.

In the last decade, specialized eating disorder units have opened at hospitals and clinics all over the country. Self-help groups provide support and referral to effective care. In 1985 the American Association of Eating Disorders Counselors formed to establish professional standards for therapists in the field. Each year more mental health care practitioners are trained to work with problems with food.

Not all anorexic and bulimic patients receive adequate care. Many still seek help at institutions where their problems are not well understood. Often these people get discouraged and drop out of treatment.

Depending on the severity of the illness, the amount of time and treatment necessary for recovery varies from a few outpatient visits to long hospitalizations and years of outpatient followup care. Because of the difficulty of correcting entrenched eating disorders, it is imperative that preventive education reach potential victims before they develop problems with food. An essential part of prevention is an attack on the cult of slenderness.

CHAPTER REVIEW

◆ ──────────VOCABULARY────────── ◆

AA/BA American Anorexia/ Bulimia Association.

ANAP National Association for Anorexia Nervosa and Associated Disorders, Inc.

Marlene Boskind-White first to describe and name bulimarexia.

Hilde Bruch early researcher in eating disorders.

William Gull first to use the term anorexia nervosa.

IAEDP International Association of Eating Disorders Professionals.

NAAS National Anorexia Aid Society.

OA Overeaters Anonymous.

psychoanalysis a form of psychotherapy that uses the theories of Sigmund Freud.

psychotherapy the psychological treatment of mental, emotional, and behaviorial disorders.

trait an inherited or acquired characteristic that is consistent, persistent, and stable.

◆ ──────FOR YOUR CONSIDERATION────── ◆

◆ Treatment for eating disorders varies a great deal in quality and availability. If you had a relative or close friend with a serious problem with food, how would you go about finding help in your neighborhood? Who would you call, and how would you check on the quality of care provided?

◆ Describe the psychological defense mechanism known as "denial" as it affects alcoholic and eating disordered persons.

◆ Many people with eating disorders are reluctant to accept treatment. List some reasons for this reluctance, and discuss what you might do to reduce it. Based on your reading up to now, what criteria would you use in recommending a person to inpatient versus outpatient treatment programs?

STEM
A Program for Recovery

This chapter will help you:

1. Know that minor problems with food can often be resolved without professional help.
2. Distinguish between minor problems and more serious disorders.
3. Subscribe to a self-help program.

◆

"Recovery meant discovering myself—having an identity that stemmed from what I am, not from what I ate, or even how I looked."

We have described disorders of appetite, eating, and weight as disorders that upset a complex equilibrium of genetic, physiological, psychological, and environmental factors. We have shown that they arise in a variety of ways by pressures operating on any or all of these aspects of a person's being. Now, as we turn to techniques for combating them, it is essential to keep in mind how individual the diseases are and how varied their causes.

In proposing a program for relief, it is wise to adopt an appropriate humility with regard to recovery. The professional and popular literature is littered with hundreds of proposals that have failed to provide lasting weight loss, programs that promise to banish anguish, diets and exercises to sculpt fresh bodies from old flesh, pills and medications to quell appetite forever, and strange garments and machines to melt fat in minutes. All appear and disappear in an endless stream.

Mass-circulated women's magazines regularly include a weight loss program of some kind. We can draw a number of conclusions from this:

1. Diets and exercise programs sell magazines and books.
2. Even though rarely correctly identified, appetite disorders must be widespread.
3. Each program must help some people in some way, thus giving credibility, but no program works for most people. If one did, it would be universally acclaimed, and deservedly so.

As you know, problems with food are stubborn disorders. They involve the entire organism—physiologically and psychologically. For most victims, they cause major disruptions in their personal and social lives, and they gnaw continually at their self-respect. To overcome them, we are proposing another diet and exercise program. We know that it had better have some unique features if it is not to share the same fate as all the others. This program is indeed unique, and this is how:

1. We address appetite first, eating second, and appearance and weight last.
2. We promise no short-term benefits.
3. We challenge you to work out your own program and leave you with complete control of your individual plan.
4. We encourage you to incorporate a changing repertoire of new ideas taken from any source, provided you are sure they are right for you.

The program is called the STEM plan. STEM is an acronym for strategy, tactics, education, and monitoring.

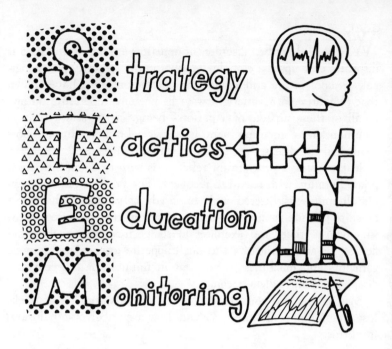

Strategy
Tactics
Education
Monitoring

The STEM plan is a guide to the big solution. If you use it, it will change your life.

The four parts of the STEM plan form an interrelated set of activities that reinforce each other in the battle against appetite disorders, or pathorexia. *Strategy* refers to a basic orientation toward healthful living. *Tactics* are the daily activities that spring from and accomplish that plan. *Education* is keeping informed about matters that are relevant to your plan. *Monitoring* is recording plans and keeping track of progress. Here is an example of how a small STEM plan might work.

Goal: To stop using food as a substitute for friendship, and reverse deterioration in health and well-being.

Strategy: Investigate local opportunities for dance and exercise classes or indoor sports programs, and make friends with people in those activities.

Tactics: Rearrange your daily schedule to create time to sample the options available. Join the most attractive programs. Then seek occasions to be social with fellow members.

Education: Check with a physician or other qualified person to discover how much exercise will be wise, given your present physical condition.

Monitoring: Keep a diary listing your plans, your progress, your impressions, and your pulse, respiration, and weight.

That is it in a nutshell. Now let us consider the parts in more detail.

The STEM concept can be used to pursue a variety of goals, so it is vital that you have a clear sense of what you want to accomplish. As you know, there are a variety of appetite disorders. The type of pathorexia you suffer from will influence how you treat it. Personal diagnosis becomes the first step in the program.

What sort of person are you, and what sort of eating disorder do you have? Are you an endomorph or a mesomorph striving to look like an emaciated ectomorph? Are you comfortable with the knowledge that you have inherited a body type from your parents that is yours for life? Do you have a nutritional history that may have made a permanent impact on your physique and metabolism? Or have you become a victim of what the educator E. H. Swengel calls "The tyranny of the impossible ideal" by believing that you can and should struggle to attain a body shape that is constitutionally beyond your reach? Please remember that a distorted image of one's body is a **common** symptom of anorexia and bulimia. What have responsible friends and family members told you about how you look?

We *will always remember the frustrated conclusion of a bulimic patient we were helping toward an appropriate diagnosis. It was clear that her mother, father, brother, two grandparents, and assorted aunts and uncles were as endomorphic a group as could be found. "My whole freaking family is infested with it!," she exploded.*

Coming to terms with our physical destiny can be a humbling experience. Like the boy who always wanted to be a policeman but reached adulthood an inch short of the minimum height, many people are desperately anxious to be slender, despite familial tendencies toward robust hips and thighs, which virtually doom the aspiring ectomorph from the start. Have you become phobic about fat and trained yourself to deny hunger and the pleasure of food in a self-destructive struggle with starvation?

Remember, 98 percent of all patients who lose weight in medically supervised programs eventually regain it. But the statistics for people who simply resolve, without professional help, to cut down on luxury edibles and who modestly boost their activity levels are far more encouraging. As many as 60 percent of them enjoy long-term success in their efforts to reduce.

Perhaps you have simply grown too fond of taking private pleasure in overeating. Or you may have become addicted to the binge and purge cycle after rigidly trying to control your appetite without success.

PROGRAM GOAL

As we have noted earlier, many people contract pathorexia by imposing a regimen of malnutrition on themselves. The STEM program could be misused to create a state of semi-starvation. If that is your goal, you will be abusing yourself and the program.

Although you may find that weight loss is a legitimate goal, many, perhaps most, pathorexics discover that their most important task is to learn to like themselves as heavier but healthier than a fashion model. If this is true for you, your task becomes learning to cope with a social environment that values the irrational idea that you can never be too thin.

We believe that many of the consequences of overeating and underexercising can be corrected, and that people who carry substantial fat do have some leeway in deciding how much they should weigh. We **do not** believe, however, that basic shapes can be altered.

Unfortunately, no formula prescribes the minimum healthy weight for any one person. We know that pathorexia occurs when weight falls below that individual minimum, and that a manageable appetite can be restored when weight is regained. But finding that lower boundary to health is a matter for personal discovery. It bears no relationship to fashion and has only a minor relationship to currently available height and weight charts.

For women of childbearing age, it is vital for health that they maintain a regular menstrual cycle when they are not pregnant or lactating (breastfeeding). To menstruate, they need a certain amount of fat, and that is one guide to minimum weight.

There is some controversy about the health of women athletes, who often stop menstruating when they are in training. Until recently, it was assumed that the exercise made up for any deficits in hormonal function, but now some experts are questioning this assumption. If you or a friend experiences athletic amenorrhea for more than four months in a row, you would be wise to consult a medical specialist. Do not let a coach's or teacher's reassurance dissuade you from getting proper medical attention.

Assessing these factors with care (that is, with care for yourself) and reflection will help you decide how much change is healthy for you and how much might further endanger your appetite control. Appendix A includes a self-scored evaluation that we use at the University of Connecticut Health Service to help people diagnose their weight and diet status. We urge you to take a few minutes to work through the questionnaire right now and then to take a few more minutes to ponder the significance of your results. Also check your responses to the questionnaire at the end of Chapter 2.

Other excellent sources of information are the books *Fat & Thin* by Anne Scott Beller (1977) and *The Dieter's Dilemma* by William Bennett and Joel Gurin (1982). We have listed these and other useful books and articles in Appendix B. Being fully educated about your own problems may well be the toughest piece of research you ever do, but it will be immensely valuable if you can clarify them sufficiently to choose the most appropriate counter-measures.

Even though the general techniques of rehabilitation are similar for all pathorexics, persons who have significant physically determined symptoms are quite different from persons whose problems are primarily psychological. Assuming that one program can treat both disorders will surely result in failure. On the other hand, it is unlikely that anyone with as complex a problem as pathorexia will ever really nail down all the various causes and consequences of his or her appetite disorder.

It has been widely noted, for example, that many bulimics have grown up in families marred by alcohol or drug abuse, or have been victims of neglect or abuse. Problems stemming from a history of ineffective parenting must be addressed directly. Counseling to help understand family issues can be undertaken in conjunction with or separate from therapy for an eating disorder. It is important, however, to acknowledge the links between the symptoms and the cause.

Do not let the search for the perfect diagnosis become an excuse for postponing the start of a therapy plan. Much effective programming for health can start immediately, with modifications and refinements introduced as you become more sophisticated.

STRATEGY

Careful strategic planning is essential to success. This is as true in personal matters as it is in politics or warfare. The fight against appetite disorder is won by people who recognize how tough a battle they are engaged in. That means reviewing a whole lifestyle, identifying the problem areas, and devising alternative behaviors that will avoid these areas. Ideally, these new activities will actively combat the temptation to abuse food.

Many pathorexics have appetite disorders that are varieties of the temptation to eat too much too often. Within that generalization, however, lies an infinite range of behaviors that make each person unique, with her or his own special problems. If you have identified yourself as a pathorexic, you too have your own patterns of food abuse, with your own ways of allowing them a place in your life.

Most pathorexics are aware of how their eating behavior deviates from healthy practice. They know the times and places that their appetite overcomes their better judgment, or when their fear of appetite leads them to take extreme countermeasures. For them, strategic planning means identifying new ways to live that minimize opportunities for those difficulties to arise.

In case you missed the message in that last paragraph, here it is again: **The strategy needed to overcome a disorder as deeply embedded as pathorexia amounts to nothing less than a new way of living.** A new way can be developed effectively using the STEM program as a guide.

For many people, their revised life is dramatically different from their old one. Changing jobs, roommates, or recreational activities are typical strategic moves. But that is not always the case.

Linda

Linda is a good example of a person who managed to change her lifestyle without any visible changes in behavior. She told us, "I've been feeling a lot better lately. I've come to accept my shape. I can't believe it; I never thought I'd be saying that!"

*Linda was bulimic when we first saw her. Then she took up dance to compensate for her bingeing. During treatment two years later, she recalled, "My original aim was to stop bingeing, to lose weight, and to have a **perfect** figure. I thought you would help me do that." She paused. "I really feel I've made this progress on my own. Now, when I dance, I concentrate on the movement, not on how many calories I'm burning.*

"I really don't have the figure for professional work, but I can teach! I'm working on my certificate now. I already teach one class, and I'll be giving another in the fall. And, you know what? I'm dating my instructor!"

An example of motivational forces associated with strategy can be drawn from work with drug addiction. Drug treatment centers have found that they can help many heroin and cocaine abusers as long as their patients live and work away from home. A return to the location where they experienced the pain of withdrawal and the relief of pain through drug use often brings back the symptoms they spent so much time and effort to lose.

There is evidence that the return of those symptoms is partly physiological. There is similar evidence with regard to appetite disorders. Exposure to situations where the symptoms were most severe causes a resurgence of unwanted appetite. The saddest aspect of this phenomenon is that home, the place where people should feel most secure, may also be the most hazardous location for the pathorexic.

Your strategies must acknowledge that being in the family kitchen, for example, may arouse a terrible craving to binge and that bingeing does not necessarily quell appetite. Otherwise, your plans will not survive the challenges of daily living.

Although pathorexia may be woven into your life because it is so closely associated with your total environment, much food abuse derives from everyday activities that are consciously distorted to provide opportunities for eating. It is very easy, for instance, to invent little victories during the day for which you can reward yourself with snacks and treats or to make routine social activities occasions for eating.

Our country's vast network of food suppliers (often aided by your family and friends) stands ready to aid and abet you in these petty indulgences. They can provide you with more to eat than you will ever need. And these same commercial interests constantly seek to give you permission to further harm yourself for their benefit.

Only people with normal appetites can resist the countless offers of food that are woven into the fabric of our culture. If you have an urge to eat that exceeds your need to eat, only a campaign that incorporates your whole way of living will effectively and permanently provide the means for a healthy life.

Keeping a safe distance from problem foods usually calls for a reorganization of the pantry and the refrigerator and a reassessment of food purchasing practices. Most people find it helpful, too, to modify their recipes by switching to low-calorie and health-oriented cookbooks.

Such changes, though easy to specify, are often difficult to initiate and maintain. Because so many eating behaviors are embedded in tradition and are inherited from loved and respected parents and grandparents (or, conversely, are adopted to ease disappointment with parents), you should anticipate a resistance to making these changes, an opposition to continuing them, and frequent temptations to abandon them. It will require your active acceptance of the entire STEM program to make your strategies stick.

Developing a strategy for living is especially difficult for the many pathorexics who have learned to be passive persons. Passivity, like eating, is another quality that is encouraged and rewarded in our society. Many people find they have fewer problems if they adopt a "go along to get along" attitude in social situations. They excuse their weakness by telling themselves they are being considerate and generous. In fact, they are letting themselves be ruled by other people's decisions, which usually means acting for other people's benefit.

Most passive, dependent people only seem peaceful. Passionate emotions that we all share are hidden from view. The hunger for love, the pressure of anger, and the empty feelings of loneliness are all present inside. These repressed emotions can find symbolic expression in eating behaviors. For example, when the love and attention that agreeableness should earn are not adequately reciprocated, dependent persons may regress to the more primitive comforts provided by cakes, cookies, and the various treats that children love.

Sometimes anger inhibited in social and familial situations may be partially released through spasms of vomiting—graphic enactments of the thought, "Such and such a person or problem really makes me sick!" or "I have to take things in, digest them, and then bring them up later. I can never react spontaneously."

To make matters worse, many heavy pathorexics have another hurdle on their path to health: their tendency to move slower and less often than their normal weight friends. Looked at in a positive light, it could be said that such people are efficient organisms, burning fewer calories per hour than the people around them. Unfortunately (as they see it), their surplus of stored fat means they can become more healthy by becoming more active.

If this is true for you, you may find that mobilizing yourself to burn energy through exercise is one of the hardest changes to make. In the long run, however, you will discover it to be a rewarding and eventually pleasurable aspect of your new lifestyle. Individuals who have reached a state of stable obesity and who no longer consume more than they expend are well advised to make increased energy expenditure their principal method of enhancing health and improving appearance.

Strengthening muscles and improving heart and lung function are the most natural ways to raise metabolic rate and trim fat tissue. Aerobic exercises such as walking, dancing, running, swimming, or cycling do not cause increases in lean tissue size, although they may increase muscle density and weight. Instead, they reintroduce you to behaviors your body is designed for but which 20th century living has minimized or eliminated.

Done in moderation, rediscovering your body's natural functions is a self-reinforcing process that gains momentum continually. Done in excess, exercise becomes an addictive, self-destructive routine that mirrors the victim's belief that they do not deserve to feel good about themselves. (Many normal and underweight pathorexics are guilty of this.)

A note on mental health. Many people who are reluctant to acknowledge emotional problems like chronic anxiety or depression "medicate" themselves by overeating. If you have a tendency to ignore or deny problems or substitute one symptom for another, competent counseling may well make the difference between the success and failure of your STEM program strategy.

If you have a tendency toward this kind of excess, you need strategies that set limits on your exercise program so you can maintain fitness and well-being without crowding out more enriching recreational activities.

The exact nature of the exercises that best meet your needs is going to be as individual as the rest of your strategy, but there are some broad guidelines that can be helpful. First, a truly effective program will be one that fits smoothly into your daily routine. If you can actually make it one of your daily responsibilities, so much the better. For people with essentially sedentary occupations, the best opportunity for putting exercise into their schedules is often on the road to work or school.

Walking, running, or cycling to and from work or to and from a strategically parked car can reverse a decline into obesity and subsequent pathorexia by tipping the energy balance into the modest deficit needed to regain health and lose unwanted pounds.

Lisa

A good example of a person who found a way to include necessary exercise in her life is Lisa, who literally halved her weight from 224 pounds in March to 112 pounds in December, when she first sought treatment from us. She had accomplished this loss by living solely on a diet product. Lisa looked sick: hollow cheeks, black eye sockets, wispy hair. She was perpetually tired, often dizzy, and had fallen victim to a succession of colds and flu.

She came to us because she was afraid she could not stop losing weight and was equally afraid of regaining it. It was the second time in 18 months that she had been this starved.

After we convinced Lisa that only refeeding could save her health, the dam burst on her appetite. We set an initial goal weight as that at which her period returned. When that happened at 145 pounds, she was gaining at the rate of 10 pounds a week! She leveled off at 185 pounds, which we discovered was her natural healthy weight and one that she could easily maintain if she got moderate exercise.

Lisa's strategy was simple. She quit her sedentary job as a cashier and went back to her old job as a waitress. She also rejoined a bowling league. Before she was able to restore herself to health, Lisa needed the educational input that taught her the hazards of attempting to have a body shape different from her natural heredity.

Some people who need to exercise to maintain health resent the fact that their friends are able to remain essentially inactive without gaining weight. It is important to remember the vast individual differences among us. We need to recognize that a few lucky people are constitutionally well adapted to an inactive life. Unfortunately, we cannot use their example to justify our own indolence.

To summarize, strategy for most people means making substantial changes in three major areas. The first is rerouting life away from unhealthful food and food-related activities while preserving and enhancing normal, pleasurable nutrition. The second is building in a daily opportunity to exercise. The third is seeking insight into and solutions for the personal weaknesses that inhibit carrying out the first two decisions.

Good strategies will introduce changes in ways that add interest and stimulation to your life rather than imposing regimens that require discipline and sacrifice. It is a central concept of the STEM program that you add more than you subtract.

As a final word on strategy, we urge you to avoid the trap of allowing a prepackaged diet plan to be your strategy. Neither books, nor organizations, nor experts can specify what you need for you, though many promise to do just that—for a fee.

There is a great temptation for people who are faced with the huge problem of pathorexia to deceive themselves into thinking that they can pay someone else for a solution. Doctors, dietitians, books, and organizations can help, but they cannot cure. Incorporating someone else's plan into your strategy may be a good idea, but making it your whole plan will ensure failure.

Nobody can tell you how to live your life. Overcoming an appetite disorder requires a complex restructuring, and you are the expert, the architect, and the contractor. You need help, but the program and its execution are yours alone.

TACTICS

Tactics are the daily implementation of strategic decisions, modified to meet the constant variations that arise in your life. A well-planned strategy creates a health-oriented lifestyle. Appropriate tactics reinforce your overall goals in innumerable minor ways that give vitality to your program and blend it into your life.

Your strategy does not merely replace unhealthy activities with healthy ones. It enriches the content of your life by helping you develop autonomy, variety, and sophistication. So tactical approaches emphasize growth, independence, and novelty in more intimate and immediate concerns. Tactics have three purposes:

they implement strategy, they combat routine responses, and they stimulate fresh awareness. Put these together and you become a more interesting person.

If you are pathorexic, your daily challenge is to find ways to keep inappropriate eating out of routine activities and to enlarge your repertoire of healthy behaviors. This challenge can best be met through a combination of planned activities and a preplanned set of responses to unanticipated events.

Planning itself can be broken into two activities: evaluating and scheduling. As you look ahead to the immediate future, you are faced with a variety of activities that you must choose among.

Many of these possibilities are so essential to your well-being that you hardly consider them to be choices: working, washing, eating, sleeping, greeting friends and family, and so on. Other daily events are clearly optional: how you dress and what you do for recreation are typical areas in which you exercise conscious choices.

To carry out your daily round of activities, you must at some point evaluate alternatives, make choices based on your judgment, and then develop a schedule that you follow.

The STEM program brings that entire process to the forefront of your attention. Creating tactics is a matter of evaluating and scheduling possible activities and using their therapeutic value as a criterion for choosing what you will do.

Accepting STEM means accepting responsibility for your life. That acceptance may reach down to the smallest of activities, especially with regard to tactics. It is quite likely that the way you link together the larger portions of your day presents major opportunities for healthy choices that can establish a style for subsequent behaviors.

For example, because of their overactive appetites, pathorexics frequently sneak a snack into breaks in their schedule. As described in Chapter 8, snacks are more likely to sharpen appetite than to suppress it. Therefore, if eating between meals can be avoided, pathorexia will be eased. The tactical response here may be to seek activities that will undermine the hazardous association between free time and eating.

Alternatives to snacks include recreational walking, shopping, reading a book or newspaper, having conversations, writing letters, knitting, or, better yet, doing something for yourself that adds another plus to your day.

Taking responsibility for your life means providing properly for your daily nutritional needs. Nobody has found a better long-term way of doing that than eating balanced meals three or four times a day. All pathorexics resist eating scheduled meals. Anorexics would just as soon not eat; the rest look upon skipping a meal as a way of building up credit that can be used in the next binge, or as compensation for previous ones.

There is no way you can regain health and still play these games with yourself. Retraining yourself to plan, prepare, and enjoy regular meals is the most important tactical change you can make.

The most effective way that healthy eating can be achieved is through adopting the OA principle, "One day at a time." Nobody with an entrenched eating disorder can ever assume that a one-time decision to reform will be powerful enough to last a lifetime. But to hold the line on health from today until tomorrow is a manageable proposition—and the most important single tactic you can employ.

Both OE and AA have helped millions of people turn their lives around through the use of this simple rule. You can use it today! Then decide tomorrow if you can use it again. Ask yourself,

"Can I eat wisely just for today?" Remember, tomorrow remains completely unknown; who knows what you might choose to do then! Make your decision for today alone.

Once you have committed yourself to a day's worth of healthy eating, one tactical problem that will arise is coping with the unexpected shocks and stresses that you have been accustomed to handling by manipulating your diet. When the stresses come, you can ask yourself "Is this worth bingeing over?" or "Is this worth starving over?", depending on the impulse you are subject to.

If you can make this crucial shift from reacting to reflecting during a crisis, you will be able to master situations that previously overwhelmed you. (Note that the question "Is this worth bingeing or starving over?" may at times get a "Yes!" answer.)

If disordered eating has been your way of coping with stress for a long time, it is all too likely that the temptation to try the old solution will sometimes be irresistible. That will not mean that your strategy needs to be changed or that your tactic of taking one day at a time has been discredited. It will simply remind you that the struggle with pathorexia is difficult and cannot always be won.

Your STEM program uses setbacks as learning opportunities. After a slip, ask yourself, "Was that worth getting sick over?" Then seek a more productive way to deal with a similar problem if it should arise in the future. Remember, because you take one day at a time, you start fresh every morning. At the beginning of their program, some people make it one hour at a time or even less when they are seriously tempted to backslide.

Like the other three segments of the STEM program, tactics requires you to shift your decision making from the flawed and obscure processes we described in Chapters 6 and 7 to the rational center of your upper brain—the part of your brain that figured out that you needed to read this book!

Ideally, your awareness of a problem should pave the way to its solution, but in practice we find that that is usually not the case. Even when unconscious forces are made conscious, they are still the same forces and they still pressure you to act in the same destructive ways. Good tacticians often seek a compromise rather than insist on victory or defeat.

A recovering pathorexic patient who has learned to stay out of harm's way by visiting her parents' home only briefly and keeping all food out of her own room, said, "I don't like the feeling that I'm not in control, that I can't have food around because if it's there I'll eat it all at once and throw up. But I **do** like the feeling that my life isn't being lived for food anymore."

It is better to lose a few battles and win the war than to experience costly victories on minor issues that drain your strength for the long campaign. Consider the example of Dave.

Dave

An example of someone who picked a poor tactic is Dave, who was overweight because his sales job required him to entertain many customers in expensive restaurants.

Dave resolved to end overindulgence once and for all! He made this decision on June 30. The following Friday, July 4, was his family's annual reunion and picnic, an event that Dave traditionally organized and cooked for.

Dave did not handle himself well at the party. He refused to cook anything he believed to be high in calories and boasted about his new lifestyle to his assembled family.

Predictably, his family thought Dave was being immature and did not hesitate to say so. In retrospect, Dave agreed with them. He felt foolish and defeated. Within days he was off his diet and back to his old eating patterns.

Many of our clients identify with Dave's dilemma.

Another example where compromise is better than confrontation is the problem of night eating, which so often afflicts people who have to study or do similar boring tasks in the evening. For most people, late evening hunger is triggered by both physical and psychological forces. Falling blood sugar pricks the appetite, and isolation and fatigue lower the resistance to temptation. If the person skipped a meal or even just skimped, earlier in the day, the urge to eat will be even more powerful.

The ensuing raid on the refrigerator is physically gratifying but emotionally confusing as pleasure and planning conflict. Often a psychic numbing results, willpower is suspended, and the person indulges in an extended binge.

Although night eating is usually portrayed as an individual problem, it is often a group phenomenon. An example is when friends get together and spontaneously opt for beer and pizza at midnight—fun while it lasts but deeply regretted the next day.

A variation on this theme common among pathorexics is the low-key binge that accompanies irksome responsibilities. Brief periods of work are punctuated by forays for snacks, typically consisting of high-calorie foods and low-calorie drinks. The intake during such an evening may well exceed the caloric total of the day's three meals, but it is consumed in such small samples that each bite seems insignificant. Such transparent self-deceptions are nevertheless enough to sabotage any number of resolutions to reform. Tactically, such occasions are not the time to take a stand against inappropriate eating. It is better to acknowledge them as special weaknesses and to move to minimize the damage.

Plan ahead and have on hand stocks of low-calorie supplies: teas, bouillon, vegetables, and fruit that you can snack on during the long hours of work. Review both your strategies and your tactics to see if you can avoid being committed to dull, appetite-provoking activities in the evenings. Opt out of a central role in preparing for feasts. Seek support from friends and family rather than boasting about your new determination to be disciplined.

Other tactical responses are needed to cope with surprise attacks on your appetite. Birthday parties and other celebrations require a repertoire of behaviors if you wish to avoid habitual food abuse without losing your friends or your self-respect. This is especially true when alcohol is being served. Only clearly established rules can survive the dulling of good judgment that alcohol induces.

An especially relevant piece of research warrants mention here. Scientists Peter Herman and Janet Polivy, who have spent many years working on the psychology of eating, found that many normal weight people claim that they are very conscious of their desire to overeat and avoid weight gain only through deliberately restrained eating.

In one experiment, such people were asked to test the flavor of ice creams after drinking small milkshakes. It was found that the more milkshakes the restrained eaters were required to consume, the more ice cream they sampled in the flavor test. The researchers were easily able to break the resolve of these restrained eaters to diet by having them drink milkshakes and so precipitate overeating.

People who reported no need to control their eating behaved in the opposite fashion: the more milkshakes they were required to drink, the less ice cream they ate.

A number of useful concepts can be inferred from this simple experiment. First, there are people, lots of them, who effectively maintain normal weight through self-restraint. Second, it is not difficult temporarily to break down that restraint by applying psychological and environmental pressure. Third, and most important, both restraint and failure can co-exist in normal weight people. In other words, **you do not have to be perfect to succeed!** Fourth, and most important, **the harder you try to be perfect, the greater is your chance of failure.**

A final note with regard to alcohol: A significant minority of overeaters are also alcohol abusers, and the two disorders have a good deal in common. Many people with a combined problem attend both AA and OA meetings. We are aware of no ongoing treatment program that can compare with the cost effectiveness or long-term success rate of these two organizations. For people who have lost control of their use of alcohol or whose appetite totally dominates their behavior, a referral to AA or OA is often the first step toward regaining control of their lives.

If you believe that you have reached that stage, call AA or OA now. Also contact by telephone or mail one of the national organizations such as AA/BA, ANAD, IAEDP, or NAAS; these groups are dedicated to providing support and therapy for people with appetite disorders. Their addresses and telephone numbers appear in Appendix B.

Do not expect this book or any other individual self-help program to provide enough insight, motivation, or support to enable you to overcome these disorders alone.

EDUCATION

As we have emphasized, coming to terms with appetite disorders usually involves acknowledging the need for major changes in living patterns. We have discussed how strategy and tactics can help you devise and maintain these changes, but a third essential ingredient for good planning is **good information**—knowing what you are about. The more you know about yourself and your behavior, the better your chances are of making wise choices that can improve your well-being.

Although this principle is almost self-evident, putting it into practice in the matter of appetite and eating disorders is not that easy. The reason is not that there is any lack of information, but that there are so many contradictory views and a great deal of misinformation and genuine confusion in both popular and scientific literature.

A consistent effort to be well informed is essential for avoiding regression to past practices. There is no way your newly formed strategies and tactics will overcome bad habits if they are not properly supported by reliable facts and figures that help you justify choosing the road to health over the rut of illness. Only when you

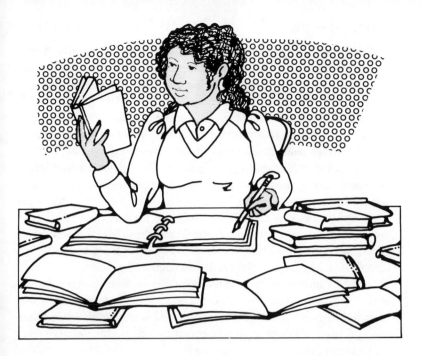

believe that you have learned something about health and about yourself will you be mentally equipped to make significant changes in your life.

How do you go about becoming better informed? Very carefully! Be aware from the start that there is more misinformation than good information available from both the print and broadcast media and in much professional-based material.

We have mentioned several books and other publications by name throughout this text. The suggested readings given at the end of the book provide an introduction to the literature that you will find helpful. Look for these references in a college or university library or at public libraries or in book stores. We urge you to read as many of these books and publications as you can find.

Popular books and magazine articles are much less reliable sources of information. They almost always present viewpoints that are too optimistic and too narrow to be considered responsible. Although developments in the field do get reported in the mass media, the doubts, questions, and qualifications that the researchers themselves express about their work are often minimized or omitted to keep the stories both exciting and brief.

Do not accept anything on trust. Rather, put new and interesting information on probation. Test it out and look for confirmation from other sources and from your own experience before incorporating it into your store of knowledge.

Read over Chapters 6, 7, and 8 once more, especially if you skimmed through them the first time. Some of the information may be a little hard to grasp fully, but you will become familiar with a lot of important scientific research.

As you inquire about psychology and physiology, nutrition and exercise, recreation and pastimes, and so become an informed person, be aware that professional disagreements exist in every field of knowledge. Forewarned is forearmed. Do not let a controversy between experts undermine your own determination to regain your personal health.

A case in point is the dispute over the toxicity of sugar. There are nutritionists who are sure sugar is harmless, whereas others regard it as positively dangerous and indict it for numerous ills and disorders. Chances are, the truth lies somewhere between the two schools of thought. While we all await the verdict, prudent pathorexics will be alert to the issue and will carefully review their use of sugar in light of their own experience with it. Bleached flour has also been indicted by some experts and cleared by others. Your own experience should be your guide.

Brian

We have found that many of our patients are very susceptible to sugar. One of our patients, Brian, told us, "When I'm abstinent I feel fine and act fine, but when I get into sugar, a tremendous anger erupts within me." Counseling helped Brian to recognize that allowing himself to feel the rush that sugar gave him put him in touch with other legitimate but suppressed appetites that he had been striving to ignore because he thought of them as weaknesses. Although he learned to accept a whole new identity, sugar remained a hazardous substance for Brian, although not so much as before he sought treatment.

Educating yourself may mean much more than simply reading books and magazine articles. It can include discovering your personal history by tracking down medical records. Begin, if you can, by talking with your parents and your grandparents about your behavior as a child, and try to distinguish between the reality and the legends about your growth and development. Concentrate on family customs and values associated with food and eating.

Other contacts with interested people and experts of all kinds can expand your awareness and understanding of your behavior (Figure 10-1). Contacts such as these may forge links between the

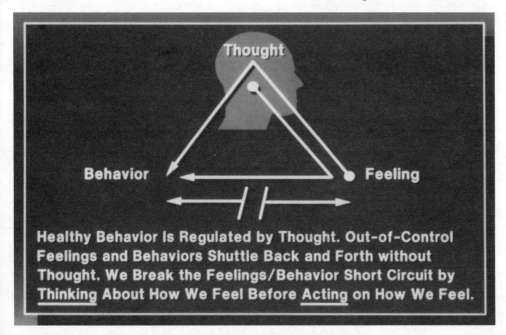

Figure 10-1. *The behavior triangle.*

four parts of the STEM program. Attending OA meetings, for example, would be both a strategic and a tactical decision, but it would also qualify as an educational experience. Learning how others cope with their symptoms can be a powerful boost for your own therapy. The same linkage occurs for strategies that include counseling or psychotherapy, or when a tactical decision to switch from coffee breaks to reading breaks leads you to new knowledge about health.

Finally, being informed is fun, and sometimes even exciting. Health maintenance and nutrition are swiftly changing fields in which new knowledge is being generated continually. Obesity and eating disorders are proving to be extraordinarily complex phenomena. Genetic, organic, and environmental components that were often neglected in the past are now being studied carefully.

Keeping abreast of advances in understanding obesity and nutrition and knowing how personally affected you may be become an absorbing pastime. And, provided you use the information judiciously, it is a valuable social asset that you can share with interested friends.

MONITORING

For many people, the toughest part of their jobs is the paperwork! Keeping accounts is boring and often seems unnecessary. Unfortunately, records are important. Monitoring is a vital component of the STEM program.

Although recordkeeping sounds dull, when you are moving in the right direction, it becomes a continuing success story, and that is not dull at all! Your diary of progress will be a powerful inducement to further progress. The more closely you monitor your behavior, the greater your incentive will be to make that behavior rewarding and to improve on past performance.

There is a second and more important reason for monitoring your behavior when you combat pathorexia: it is a great help in raising your conscious awareness of what you are doing. The central disorder in pathorexia is that your instincts no longer correspond with your needs—what you want to do makes you ill. It therefore becomes essential that you take charge of your instincts and that you accept more responsibility for your behavior. As for administrators everywhere, that means you increase the paperwork.

So what do we mean by monitoring? There are two major processes involved: recording what you intend to do and recording what you have done and how you feel about your performance. When they are not blocking out their feelings about food, people with severe eating disorders often feel guilty and upset about everything that goes into their mouths. Because they are so prone to abusing food, they perceive all their eating as wrong.

A safe way out of this difficulty is to adopt a technique pioneered by OA. What you do is **commit** at the beginning of the day to eating an appropriate selection and quantity of food. You are then free to enjoy thoroughly three or four guilt-free meals. All other foodstuffs are off limits, so there is no point in even thinking about them. Research studies have shown that the principle is a good one.

Planning ahead and specifying precisely what you regard as acceptable behavior greatly enhances the likelihood of your staying within those healthy limits. It is important when you do this that you plan for an adequate and nutritionally complete menu. If you plan too sparse a menu for the day, there will come a moment of self-pity accompanied by a spasm of unscheduled overeating.

At first, most people need help in figuring out their food plan. The great temptation is to commit too little. A dietitian or an OA sponsor can be of immense value in this task, but do not give up the decisions to your helper. With guidance, make up your own plan.

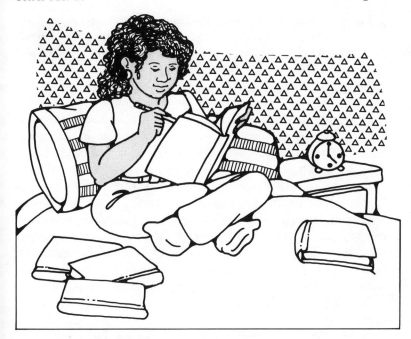

This principle can be applied to more than just eating. You will be far more likely to complete your exercises or your studies if you keep these activities comfortably within your abilities and if you schedule them ahead of time. Good management requires good planning, so set healthy, attainable goals.

In the journal that develops from monitoring your progress, devote some space to notes and comments about your strategy and tactics. Here is where you commit to writing what you want to accomplish, the long-term plans you have for achieving these goals, and the dozens of tricks and techniques that can help on a daily basis.

Also record any other information that may be pertinent for you: facts and statistics about nutrition and health, personal statistics, even a wish list of desirable rewards and treats you can celebrate with. A working journal soon takes on a life of its own. It becomes the natural place to file phone numbers, friends' birthdates, and anything else you need to have at your fingertips.

As you build up a store of information and become accustomed to adding to and drawing from your journal, you will enormously reinforce the rational powers of your brain because recordkeeping is a rational process.

Do not assume or be concerned that monitoring might transform you into a cold, logical being. Just the reverse is more likely to occur. You will become emotionally freer, more relaxed, and able to enjoy more fully the good things in life as you lose the nagging fear that you are an inept, undisciplined failure at life's important tasks.

Having a plan and sticking to it gives you confidence in yourself, and having a journal in which to confide your hopes, apprehensions, successes, and disappointments helps you validate your emotions and accept them for what they are—the color and spice of your life, a daily reminder of your unique nature.

Almost as important as looking ahead is keeping track of what is actually happening to you. This will be the enjoyable part of monitoring. A "mood and food" diary in which you record everything that makes a day notable will quickly become a fascinating account of progress. Although, for a pathorexic person, changes in eating behaviors will be emphasized in the record, a journal gains depth, character, and insight only when emotional matters are included also.

Self-knowledge requires self-examination and reflection. Confiding regularly in a diary is one of the better ways to achieve this. Inevitably, you will refer repeatedly to the issues that give you the most trouble. As the record grows, it will become harder to ignore or excuse patterns of failure, and it will become easier to discover how these patterns operate. The relationships among your environment, your appetites, your emotions, and your behaviors will be clarified. With this knowledge, you can take steps toward a more self-directed, autonomous lifestyle. You will no longer see yourself as a victim of circumstances.

Your journal will be an effective tool only if you use it. That means you need to read over frequently what you have written to compare the present with the past. Doing so permits you to engage in a dialogue with yourself about the most important matters in your life. When your journal includes candid, unvarnished, and unedited opinions about your strengths (be sure not to forget these) and your weaknesses, you greatly increase your awareness of yourself.

If, despite this feedback, you find yourself continuing to behave in ways that mystify and depress you, think about professional counseling as a means of gaining greater insight and control. Working with a psychotherapist on these problems will enable you to receive objective feedback. Together, you will be able to devise a more powerful STEM program.

Because your journal is the active center of your entire STEM program, it is important that you treat it with respect. The more you invest in your journal, the better it will serve you. Begin by purchasing a quality hardcover journal, something that will look good and will wear well. After all, it is going to be volume one of a very important autobiography! The design, size, and number of pages can reflect your personal preference, but do not skimp on quality. Your story is too valuable to be committed to a junky notebook.

To conclude this chapter, we want to emphasize a theme we have sounded throughout this book. We want to remind you that pathorexia is a stubborn, hard-to-correct disorder, but that its progress can be halted and held in remission through a far-reaching revision of customary behaviors.

STEM AS A CONTINUING PROJECT

Arresting pathorexia will change your life, but you must change your life to arrest pathorexia. Because this is so, it is essential to think of the STEM program as a continuing project that has neither a timetable nor a termination

Remember that nothing worthwhile is accomplished without error. Little worth doing is done right the first time. Testing your program by finding out what strategies, tactics, and recordkeeping methods do not work for you is part of the process of discovering what **does** work.

Recognizing the importance of trial and error in forming your program is a giant step toward undermining the perfectionism so prevalent among pathorexics. Work your program a step at a time, gathering strength and confidence as you go. But anticipate setbacks, and refuse to be discouraged simply because you temporarily slip back into an all-too-familiar rut.

One final word: **share your program.** Look for a person or persons who will endorse your commitments and support your efforts, especially when you experience failure. If you feel that you cannot confide in a friend or cannot afford a therapist, yet you need more support, call OA.

OA has over 20 years of experience working with the symptoms of pathorexia. Its members have lots of respect for the disease and a record of achievement that gives hope to even the most discouraged. Restored by the support of understanding people, you can return to your program once more, gain another day of healthy behavior and a further increment of self-respect.

BASIC PRINCIPLES FOR RECOVERY

Finally, here is a list of basic principles for recovery.

1. A. **There is no lasting relationship between a sense of well-being and being overfed and overweight or being underweight and malnourished.** A central myth of our materialistic culture is that consumption can make you happy. The central myth of eating disorders is that weight loss brings fulfillment. Since gaining and losing weight are America's favorite pastimes, you can get plenty of reinforcement for these myths. The difference between America's pastimes and your compulsive eating, anorexia, or bulimia is a matter of degree.

   B. Remember that pathorexics play for keeps! Gourmands and dieters, on the other hand, play for fun. Sure, they like to eat and lose weight, but only food abusers are willing to risk their health in these pursuits. The rest of us quit before problems get out of hand. This is especially true of dieting and weight loss. Pathorexics think other people are also deadly serious about their weight. They do not realize that most of us talk a lot more than we act.

2. **In achieving a clear sense of personal identity, what you are is more important than how you look.** Look around you, look at people just a bit older and at people who are 20 years older than you are. Let's face it, not many of us are beautiful. And not all beautiful people are thin. We like our friends for how they live, not how they look.

3. **No one gets out of the binge and purge cycle without relearning to eat a regular, healthy diet.** Skipping meals, eating too little, or trying to stay underweight are guarantees of failure. It isn't easy to quit food abuse. Your body adapts to eating disorders. Your entire digestive tract from top to bottom must readjust to normal eating. In the early phase of recovery you may experience a whole array of discomforts: swollen glands, bloated feelings, constipation, excess appetite, and, scariest of all, fast weight gain, are all possible. If you have abused laxatives, you may have to taper off slowly so your body can learn to do without them. During this time, keep in mind that all the pains and changes are part of recovery, and they do not last long. You can and will return to normal eating if you want to, and if you keep working at it.

4. **Purging—especially vomiting—is the mechanism that keeps the bulimic cycle going.** This is also one thing you have real control over. It is easier to say no to purging than

to bingeing, and if you stop the purge, the binges will taper off—not immediately, but after a few days. As soon as your digestive system learns it has food to work with, it will stop arousing your appetite. Have patience while your body recovers.

5. **For women of childbearing age, regular menses are vital for long-term health.** If weight loss or excess exercise has affected your periods, the best measure of regained health is renewed menstruation. Again, this may be a bit scary, but it goes with being adult and female. If after thinking about this awhile, you're still uncomfortable, it is probably time to talk to a counselor.

6. **Do not suffer alone if self-help fails.** Talk things over with a dietitian or a mental health professional who is well informed about eating disorders. Or go to an OA meeting. You are not going to shock them, and they are not going to embarrass you. They will help you assess your situation and work with you toward recovery. So don't hesitate. And don't stay with a therapist or sponsor that you think is incompetent. Find someone who knows what you are talking about and to whom you can relate.

SUMMARY

STEM is a self-help program you can use. Effective self-help involves four processes: strategic plans, tactics, education, and monitoring—STEM, for short.

Strategy means thinking out a plan for your life for the next year or so, deciding what would be practical and possible for you. Set some realistic goals regarding your health, physique, activities, and achievements that are in line with your personality, not with other people's hopes and expectations.

Tactics are the day-to-day activities that help you achieve your goals. For example, if night eating binges are a problem for you, plan to eat a legitimate snack or supper about 11 p.m., and follow it with another activity (preferably one with other people) until you go to bed. If you have gotten into a habit of heading for the bathroom after dinner, find something else to do while your meal digests. Schedule healthy activities into your day so you do not need to rely on just willpower to get you through.

Education is self-discovery. Instead of blotting out thoughts and feelings with food, get to know yourself and your behaviors. Use this book and the reading list at the end of it for in-depth knowledge about food abuse. Come to terms with your own strengths and weaknesses. Reflect on your family history. Get some vocational counseling. Look for honest feedback from friends and people you respect. Get a better feeling for who **you** are. Then apply the knowledge to your strategies.

Monitoring is keeping track of progress. If you are serious about changing your behavior, you need to keep track of what you are doing. Use a journal to record your strategy, tactics, thoughts, and feelings about yourself. Then write down food-related activities each day, and highlight with contrasting colors the good and the bad behaviors. Do not expect overnight success, but do look for a noticeable shrinking of the "bad" if you are going to tackle your problem alone. If you cannot see progress after a month of working on your problem, get professional help.

CHAPTER REVIEW

♦ ————————FOR YOUR CONSIDERATION———————— ♦

♦ In a small group, set yourselves the task of creating healthier and more enjoyable relationships with food. Outline a STEM program that would be helpful for people of your age, in your situation.

♦ Individually, revise the program to meet your personal needs more effectively. Who would you need to discuss your plan with in order to put it into effect? Develop some discussion points that you might use in talking over your STEM plan. Anticipate the major obstacles to implementing your STEM plan, and consider ways to overcome them, or accommodate to them.

APPENDIX A

Self-Evaluation Exercise

This appendix includes a self-evaluation tool that we use at the University of Connecticut Health Service. *Calorie Counters are Losers* was prepared for patients who consult the university nutritionist. We have found it to be useful and thought provoking. It is especially helpful for people who are planning a STEM program.

CALORIE COUNTERS ARE LOSERS*

We live in a culture that is preoccupied with being slim. Most people think that the fatter you are, the more carelessly you've been eating; and that the skinnier you are, the less you've been eating, the more self-control you have. This is not always true. This line of thinking leads to poor eating habits, guilt, unhappiness, and even discrimination against fat people.

The truth is, every body is different. Most people fall into three main categories. To find out what category your body is in, take the following quiz:

1. How long have you considered yourself "too fat"?
   A. Only in the last year
   B. Since puberty
   C. Since early childhood

2. What is the most "overweight" you have ever been?
   A. 5-10 pounds
   B. 10-25 pounds
   C. 25-50 pounds
   D. over 50 pounds

3. How often have you been within five pounds of the weight you would like to weigh?
   A. Until recently
   B. Occasionally after dieting
   C. Rarely, even after dieting
   D. Never

4. How many other people in your biological family are fat?
   A. No one else
   B. One parent or a sibling
   C. Both parents
   D. One or more parents and siblings

(Exercise Continued)

5. Which of the statements below best describes the kind of eating behavior you worry most about and want to change?
   A. When my friends are eating snacks, I can't resist joining them
   B. I frequently eat large meals
   C. I nibble constantly between meals
   D. Diet for a few days or weeks but then go on an uncontrolled food binge

6. How often in the past five years have you tried to lose weight?
   A. Never
   B. Once
   C. Several times
   D. I'm always trying to lose weight

Now evaluate your score using the accompanying table. The number of points for each response is at the intersection of the rows and columns corresponding to each response. Total your score and then identify which group you probably belong to. (If you score near the border between groups, read the information pertaining to both groups.)

*Written by Maryann Morris, M.S., R.D., and Vivian Mayer. Used with permission.

QUESTIONS	A	B	C	D
1	1	2	3	—
2	1	2	3	5
3	1	3	4	4
4	1	3	4	5
5	1	1	2	4
6	1	1	2	2

Basically slim (total score 6-12). You have been slim or of average weight most of your life. A recent change in your lifestyle has resulted in less physical exercise or more opportunities to eat high-calorie foods than before. You may have gained 10 pounds and want to "get back in shape."

Chronic dieter (total score 13-17). You've never been so fat as to have to buy your clothes in special stores. But those few **extra** pounds keep nagging at you. Lately you may be finding it harder and harder to keep them off.

Chronic dieter plus (total score 18 or greater). Unless you stick to a low-calorie diet, you tend to be fat. You may have been fat since early childhood or since adolescence. You may have tried many times to lose weight. Each attempt ultimately failed and left you fatter than ever.

FOR EVERYONE   The special needs of each group are discussed later; these general
                          suggestions apply to everyone.

1. A well-balanced diet that is sufficient in calories, high in
   fresh produce, and low in refined sugar, processed food,
   etc., is good for nearly everyone. There should be no "forbidden foods." You should never deliberately keep yourself
   hungry.

2. Supply yourself with minimally processed foods to snack on:
   whole grain breads and muffins, fresh fruit, and vegetables.

3. Make room in your life for nonfood-oriented activities that
   you enjoy.

4. Exercise should be something you enjoy. If you don't enjoy
   your present form of exercise, try something else.

5. Avoid artificial sweeteners and special diet foods. These
   foods interfere with your natural appetite-regulating system.

6. Fatness is not a sure sign of overeating. Careful studies have
   shown that the calorie intakes of fat and slim people in
   many cases fall within the same range.

7. Dieting may make you temporarily slimmer, but it has some
   consequences that tend to make you fatter in the long run:
   (1) The longer you go with insufficient calories, the
   stronger the urge is to binge, especially on sugary foods. (2)
   The longer you go with insufficient calories, the more efficient your metabolism becomes. Ultimately, you may get as
   many calories out of an apple as a typical nondieter gets
   out of a piece of apple pie. The result: every time you stop
   dieting you gain back more than you lost.

8. We live in a culture with a heavy investment—both financially and emotionally—in the idea that the average mature body is too fat. Hence, you feel real pain when you
   look in the mirror. Given the types of food propaganda we
   face in our society, it is helpful to be conscious of how you
   eat, and to make deliberate choices. It is not helpful to be
   preoccupied with food.

You may not have been told these things before, but that is
because people only told you things that would keep you trying to
lose weight.

For one week, substitute a piece of fresh fruit for your ordinary sweet snacks and desserts. Have fresh fruits and vegetables on hand for snacking.

Eat slowly, eat the main course, and do not limit yourself solely to salads and vegetables at meal times. Carbohydrates and proteins in moderate quantities are necessary for optimal health.

Eat three meals daily at regular times. Structure your meals so there is a beginning and an end.

If you cook for yourself, decrease amounts of fat in food being cooked, but don't eliminate fat altogether. Fat adds nutrition and tends to make people feel full.

Remember that a few extra pounds gained by careless eating should come off easily but gradually if you don't try to force them. If these small changes don't make you slimmer, relax. It is natural to gain a little weight as you mature. Recent evidence suggests that a little extra weight (compared with current fashion) actually improves your health.

If You Scored Basically Slim

These groups are very similar. People who score in these groups have been worrying about their weight for a long time. The main difference is the amount of weight they've been worrying about.

If you are a chronic dieter, regardless of your size, you probably have seen the suggestions for group one many times. You don't need them now. In fact, your nutrition and metabolism may have been changed through frequent dieting so that suggestions that involve eating less are irrelevant or even harmful to you.

If You Scored Chronic Dieter or Chronic Dieter Plus

If you think you're in real danger of becoming very fat, you're right! Only the danger comes from where you least expect it. It comes not from the extra piece of cake, but from dieting.

To understand this, go back to the section For Everyone, and reread points 6, 7, and 8. Whatever you do about your weight, you must take these facts into account.

If Your Score Was Around 13-17

Guilt—undeserved—may be your biggest problem. Being fat is not a fault. Even if you think of yourself as a compulsive eater, such problems are not a fault. In fact, similar eating behaviors have been created in laboratory animals by keeping them on low-calorie diets.

The same rules of good nutrition that apply to slim people apply to you. You should not short change yourself of any nutrients, including calories.

If You Scored Over 17

HAS WORRYING ABOUT YOUR WEIGHT AFFECTED YOUR NUTRITION AND SELF-RESPECT?

Please take the following quiz:

7. How do you feel when you eat something extra, like a dessert or high-calorie snack, that you were not planning to eat?
   A. I enjoy it
   B. I enjoy it, with regrets
   C. I enjoy it, but feel very guilty and angry at myself afterwards
   D. I feel out of control and unreal

8. Which of the statements below best describes the way you feel about the exercise or active sport you engage in (or if you don't do any, how you feel when people tell you you should)?
   A. I do it for fun
   B. I get tired of it, but keep it up for health reasons
   C. My major reason is to stay slim or to lose weight
   D. I feel forced to exercise because my body embarrasses me

9. Which of the statements below best describes the pattern of your calorie intake?
   A. Almost the same from day to day
   B. Once in awhile I overeat, but I make up for it carefully
   C. Periods of dieting that may last for days or weeks, then periods of bingeing on food
   D. I overeat, then make myself vomit or take laxatives to stay slim

10. Have you ever received psychological counseling to help you lose weight?
    A. No
    B. No, but I've thought about it
    C. Yes

SCORING	A	B	C	D
7	1	2	4	5
8	1	3	4	4
9	1	2	4	5
10	1	2	3	—

If you scored near or above 11, you may be losing a lot more than weight. Information in this book can help you combat narrow-minded social attitudes. But please keep in mind that yours is a societal problem, not just a personal problem.

1. A lot of other people struggle with eating and weight. Ask your local counseling center to help you organize fat consciousness-raising groups that are separate from weight loss groups. Such groups provide positive, constructive insights and solutions.
2. It may be difficult for you to re-establish a sense of nutritional balance. You may lose weight or gain weight. Be patient with yourself. You're allowed to make mistakes.
3. Celery and other raw vegetables are excellent munchies for well-fed people, but they are no substitute for adequate calories. Try fruit, cheese, nuts, etc., especially if you have been on a low-calorie diet for a long time.
4. As you add to your wardrobe, buy new clothes with an emphasis on comfort and ease of movement.
5. Seek out people and activities that reinforce your sense of your own intelligence, your good personality, or your other abilities. You are more than a body to be judged by other people.

Remember that you have the option to either continue the losing struggle OR to learn respect and live in your body whether or not its natural size is fashionable.

TO HELP YOU START WINNING

THE WINNER'S BOX

There's a place for everyone here no matter what your size. A balanced diet, sufficient calories, and exercise you enjoy are winning strategies for nutritional balance, health, and self-confidence.

APPENDIX B

Additional Sources of Assistance

Many local and at least four national organizations exist to help victims of pathorexia. If you live in an urban or suburban area, you can almost surely find support and therapy through listings in your telephone book. Community mental health centers can be located under "Social Service Organizations" in the yellow pages. Most university health services have enough experience with appetite disorders to enable them to refer you for help even if you are not a student. State mental health associations often have listings of qualified therapists.

The two major self-help organizations, Overeaters Anonymous (OA) and Alcoholics Anonymous (AA), are listed in most large telephone directories, or you can find them by calling directory assistance in a large city near your home. These groups welcome initial inquiries by telephone and will help you make arrangements to attend a meeting by providing a sponsor and often a ride, if you need one. Their national headquarters are listed below.

The following national organizations will also put you in touch with local sources of support.

The American Anorexia/Bulimia Association
(formerly The American Anorexia Nervosa Association)
133 Cedar Lane
Teaneck, NJ 07666
Telephone (201) 836-1800

The National Anorexia Aid Society
P.O. Box 29461
Columbus, OH 43216
Telephone (614) 846-6810

The National Association of Anorexia Nervosa and Associated Disorders
P.O. Box 271
Highland Park, IL 60035
Telephone (312) 831-3438

The National Association to Aid Fat Americans, Inc.
P.O. Box 43
Bellerose, NY 11426
Telephone (516) 352-3120

Overeaters Anonymous
3730 Motor Avenue
Los Angeles, CA 90034
Telephone: Check local directories

Alcoholics Anonymous
P.O. Box 459
Grand Central Station
New York, NY 10017
Telephone: Check local directories

International Association of Eating Disorders Professionals
(formerly American Association of Eating Disorders Counselors)
34213 Pacific Coast Highway
Suite E
Dana Point, CA 92629
Telephone: (714) 248-1150

SUGGESTED READINGS

Books

Alberti, R. E., and M. L. Emmons. *Your Perfect-Right: A Guide to Assertive Behavior.* San Luis Obispo, California: Impact, 1970. The classic text on gaining assertiveness skills.

Beattie, Melody. *Codependent No More.* Center City, Minnesota: Hazelden, 1987. Guidance for disengaging from a relationshp with an addicted person.

Beller, A. S. *Fat and Thin.* New York: Farrar, Straus & Giroux, 1977. An original, scholarly, and readable text.

Bennett, William, and Joel Gurin. *The Dieter's Dilemma: Eating Less and Weighing More.* New York: America Books, Inc., 1982. A fine and readable explanation of the problems with dieting. The best single source of information on dieting and weight loss.

Black, Claudia. *It Will Never Happen to Me.* Denver, Colorado: M.A.C., 1981. For children and adult children of alcoholics.

Boskind-White, Marlene, and William C. White. *Bulimarexia: The Binge/Purge Cycle.* New York: W. W. Norton, 1983. Expert writing on overcoming eating disorders by learning assertiveness and gaining self-esteem.

Bruch, Hilde. *Eating Disorders.* New York: Basic Books, Inc., 1973. The first modern text, now a classic.

Bruch, Hilde. *The Golden Cage: The Enigma of Anorexia.* Cambridge, Massachusetts: Harvard Press, 1978. A brief version of her earlier work, geared to a lay reader.

Cauwels, Janice M. *Bulimia: The Binge-Purge Compulsion.* Garden City, New York: Doubleday and Company, Ltd., 1983. An excellent overview with a detailed account of some treatment programs.

Chernin, Kim. *The Obsession: Reflections on the Tyranny of Slenderness.* New York: Harper and Row, 1981. A very personal series of essays on femaleness and femininity.

Ernsberger, P. and P. Haskew. *Rethinking Obesity: An Alternative View of Its Health Implications.* New York: Human Sciences Press, 1988.

Keys, A., J. Brozek, A. Henschel, O. Mickelsen, and H. L. Taylor. *The Biology of Human Starvation.* Minneapolis: University of Minnesota Press, 1950. A two-volume classic that is the source of much information about the effects of food deprivation.

Keys, A. *Seven Countries: A Multivariate Analysis of Death and Cardiac Disease.* Cambridge, Mass.: Harvard University Press, 1980. A renowned expert explodes myths about disease, death, and weight.

Kinoy, Barbara P. (Ed.). *"When Will We Laugh Again": Living and Dealing with Anorexia and Bulimia.* New York: Columbia University Press, 1984. Prepared by the American Anorexia/Bulimia Association to help victims and their families.

Levenkron, Steven. *The Best Little Girl in the World.* New York: Warner Books, 1979. A short, poignant novel about anorexia.

Levine, M. P. *How Schools Can Help Combat Student Eating Disorders,* National Education Association, Washington, DC, 1987.

Orbach, Suzie. *Fat is a Feminist Issue, II.* New York: Berkeley Publishing Corp., 1982. A forceful feminist perspective on society's impact on women's identities.

Orbach, Suzie. *Hunger Strike.* New York: W. W. Norton, 1986. A feminist therapist's view of treatment for anorexia.

Polivy, Janet, and C. Peter Herman. *Breaking the Diet Habit: The Natural Weight Alternative.* New York: Basic Books, Inc., 1983. A book on the dangers of dieting by the researchers who discovered them.

Schoenafielder, Lisa, and Barb Weiser (Ed.). *Shadow on a Tightrope: Writings by Women on Fat Oppression.* 1983. Spinsters/Aunt Lute Book Company, P.O. 410687, San Francisco, CA 94141. A fresh, strident, often shocking book on being fat in a fat-phobic society.

Weiss, Lillie, Melanie Katzman, and Sharlene Wolchik. *You Can't Have Your Cake and Eat it Too: A Program for Controlling Bulimia.* 1986. R & E Publishers, Saratoga, CA 95070. A practical guide for overcoming bulimic symptoms.

The International Journal of Eating Disorders. John Wiley & Sons, 605 Third Avenue, New York, NY 10158. The journal in which professionals publish their views and research findings. Available in university and medical libraries.

Journals

Big Beautiful Women. Encino, CA 91316

Radiance. Box 31703, Oakland, CA 94604

Fashion Magazines for Heavy Women

INDEX